# SHE

## has breast cancer

DANICA BUNCH

This book is dedicated to Ava and Lui, the loves of my life.

You were born perfect. All I have given you as your mama is the gift of knowing and feeling love. You know who you are from the people you came from. You know your values and what we stand for in our family. This knowledge will always be with you, holding strong like a scaffold for your life. You can come back to this whenever you need, and you will always find the answers to solve the challenges you face.

Keep your hearts beating out this energy and these values always. Trust your knowing.

You are amazing and I love you more than anything.

That love will always be with you, to the moon and back.

- Love Mama

# About the Author

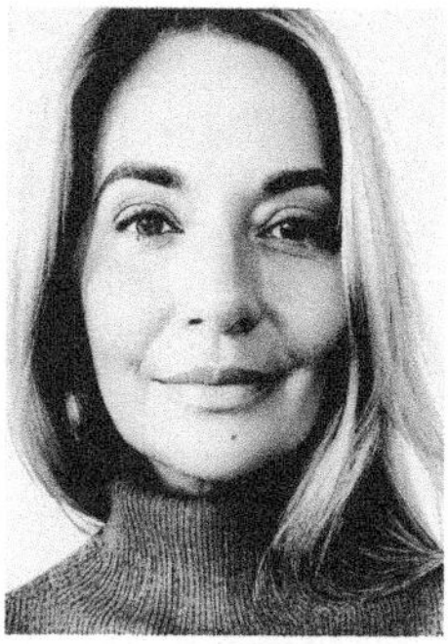

Danica Bunch is a Public Relations and Strategic Communications professional with an acumen for business strategy, crisis management leadership support and coaching. Danica is a strong networker and influencer, adept at building relationships that enhance her effectiveness in achieving outcomes for her clients.

Personally, Danica is a mother of two, old ballerina and spin class tragic. Her life has taken a turn with a recent health crisis and she is pivoting her business to include being an advocate for fundamental change in women's health. She is author of the "She. Has Breast Cancer", where she has turned her 20 years of training and craft and applied the same framework to regain control, face and understand the concept of uncertainty, recognise the impact on identity and to reach a place of strength and resilience.

# Contents

# Introduction

A breast cancer diagnosis can be overwhelming, and a woman facing this challenge needs all the support she can get. Because that support is too often lacking, I have written this book to provide practical guidance to empower women to reframe negative messaging around their diagnosis and to build the resilience that will help them to take control of their own well-being. I do not diminish the seriousness of the diagnosis, but I do explain that breast cancer is treatable. I offer unique perspective on the practical strategies and tools familiar to crisis communication used in industry and business are adapted specifically to help women, and the friends and families who support them, to navigate a breast cancer diagnosis with confidence and strength. I have drawn on my own raw story to show breast cancer patients how they can reframe damaging negative messages they may receive, promote resilience, and become active participants throughout their treatment journey from the day they are diagnosed. My book directly addresses breast-cancer patients, but caregivers will find it useful and indeed, there is much to inspire and empower any woman seeking to find strength, resilience, and hope in the face of a crisis. I provide insights and guidance based on my own experience to help you cope with the challenges ahead. I know first-hand the challenges women face when they receive a life-changing diagnosis. The waiting rooms I sat in during my diagnosis were surreal and haunting. Everywhere I looked, there were women of all ages, silently facing the same devastating diagnosis. The pink charities' PR machine promised so much support, but here we were, sitting in a sterile room, waiting for the next step with no support in sight. It was hard not to feel a sense of shared fate with these women.

As I reflect on my experiences, I've come to realise that breast cancer does not discriminate based on age. While I initially felt a deep sense of solidarity with the younger women in those waiting rooms, I now understand that breast cancer affects women of all ages. My intention in sharing my story is to reach out to all women who have faced or are currently facing breast cancer, regardless of age.

I became aware of how many women are denied early access to diagnosis simply because they're deemed too young to be at risk. I felt a deep sense of connection with these women that fuelled my determination to find a way to support us all and I decided to write a book for all women in all the waiting rooms. I aimed to provide a practical guide to help women facing breast cancer to actively engage in their treatment journey. By sharing my story and experiences, I wanted to offer hope and empowerment.

A breast cancer diagnosis affects more than just your physical health. Everything familiar and predictable is turned on its head. Fear, anxiety, and uncertainty take hold as you navigate the waters of emotional upheaval while juggling medical appointments and assessing treatment options.

It's important to remember that you are not alone. Many women have been in your shoes and have come out the other side stronger and more resilient than before. You, too, have the strength and resilience to face this challenge head-on and create a future full of possibility and potential.

And it's important to have the tools and strategies to navigate a personal crisis and that's why this book is essential for you, the woman who is facing breast cancer diagnosis. Think of this book as a roadmap. Each chapter contains practical strategies and tools for understanding the impact of a personal crisis on your identity, for embracing the power of self-care, and for finding joy and meaning.

But this book is more than just a collection of strategies and tools. My story is a reminder that you are part of a community of women who will support and uplift you. As a source of hope and inspiration, *She Has Breast Cancer* will remind you of your own inherent worth and strength.

It will show you how to:

- recognise a crisis and how crises typically play out.
- regain control using tried and tested communication tools.
- refute unhelpful and damaging labels.
- reframe your diagnosis in order to empower yourself.
- build a team around you.
- return to the new normal stronger than ever.

Through reading my journey, you will discover how to navigate this crisis with grace and courage. By means of practical exercises and tools, you will learn to embrace uncertainty, prioritise self-care, navigate the healthcare system, reject the cancer clichés and create a future full of possibility and hope. The term "cancer cliché" refers to commonly used phrases or expressions that have become overused or predictable when discussing cancer. These clichés often lack originality and fail to capture the full complexity and individuality of each person's cancer experience. It's time to reject the clichés and fight those aspects of the system that define you in terms your diagnosis or label you a victim. You can take ownership of your life and your future.

One of the essential things to keep in mind during this challenging time is good communication. It's at the heart of the issue. The kind of open and honest communication you will demand from those in the medical field also applies to interactions with loved ones and colleagues as you find the support you need. And communication with your medical team will empower you to make informed decisions about your treatment and care and to advocate for your health and well-being.

It's easy to neglect self-care when things are difficult but it's a priority in a time of crisis because it is essential to your well-being. Self-care can look different to different people. It can be as simple as taking time for a walk-in nature, practising yoga, meditating, or indulging in a favourite hobby.

It's also essential to remember that personal crises can happen to anyone, and they take many forms. It's not just a breast cancer diagnosis that can turn your world upside down. It is my hope that the strategies and tools contained in this book will help you navigate other crises you may encounter, whether they are personal or professional. By embracing uncertainty, by finding your own strength and resilience to create a positive future, you will unlock your power to navigate any crisis with grace and courage.

To summarise, as a road map this book offers practical strategies and tools to help you find the strength and resilience to embrace uncertainty, prioritise self-care, navigate the healthcare system, reject cancer clichés, and create and plan for a future of possibility and hope.

Through my own journey of coming to terms with breast cancer, I've come to understand deeply the power of resilience and of embracing uncertainty. I've learned how to find moments of joy and meaning in the darkest times and to discard the labels others have put on me. I offer practical strategies and tools to help you do the same. The book will illustrate how, in rejecting the cancer cliché and resisting the system, we can each of us take ownership of our lives, and create a world that is more accepting, empathetic, and kind.

# Chapter One:
# My Crisis

***"The Chinese use two brush strokes to write the word 'crisis.' One brush stroke stands for danger: the other for opportunity"***

- John F. Kennedy

*She Has Breast Cancer* is grounded in my own experience of the life-altering crisis that is a breast cancer diagnosis. I'll take your hand and guide you as you learn why you're experiencing certain feelings and emotions. I'll explain, step by step, real-world strategies that will empower you to understand and reframe the crisis you face and be empowered to actively respond to it.

Businesses invest in crisis management and planning for good reasons. But many of us, no matter how experienced and effective we are in juggling our complex lives, are ill-prepared to deal with the kind of devastating crisis that can derail us in an instant. Why do we as women not see ourselves as the CEOs of our lives and manage them accordingly?

My crisis started in late November 2022. I was living my best life. My business and career were taking off. My children were becoming more independent every day, and I was looking at the year ahead with anticipation and excitement. I live in a regional area, Central West NSW. I own and run a PR Agency and it involves quite a lot of travel. It's the best of both worlds. I'd been working in Melbourne for a week, and everything had gone well. It was Friday night and I'd been to dinner and drinks with colleagues. I had returned to my hotel room feeling on top of the world. I was excited and looking forward to seeing my kids the next day and returning to mummy time. I felt bulletproof, invincible as I stood in my bathroom naked, brushing my teeth. Then I noticed a slight indentation in my right breast. I passed it off as a mark from my clothes, but it was still there the next day.

My mum had had breast cancer three years earlier, in the first year of the COVID-19 pandemic in 2020. Of course, I researched whether I should be tested. I had just turned 40. When I spoke to some experts and breast cancer agencies, they said, "No, you're low risk. At your age, it's highly unlikely, and the fact your mother was over 70 makes it even more unlikely. Can you feel anything?" "No," I replied. "So, there's no need to be tested." I'm sure the pressures of the pandemic influenced this advice.

With my knowledge of my mother's experience, I made an appointment with my General Practitioner for Tuesday, four days after I had first noticed the indentation. He was wonderful. He couldn't feel much, but he insisted I have a mammogram. However, the experts' opinion was still loud in my head. Let's face it; I have the most petite ballerina boobs in the world. It seemed unbelievable that they could develop breast cancer.

My GP scheduled a mammogram for the following day. A mammogram is a type of imaging test that uses low-dose X-rays to examine the breasts for signs of cancer. Although not much was detected, I insisted on an ultrasound, a test that uses sound waves to create images of the breast tissue. I knew ultrasounds are better than mammograms at detecting small lumps and yes, the test did reveal a lump. This was followed by a core biopsy, a procedure that involves removing a small sample of tissue from the suspicious area for laboratory testing. As I waited for the results, I felt anxious and scared. I knew that not all lumps or changes in breast tissue mean cancer, but I couldn't shake off the fear. When I received the news that it was cancer, I was devastated.

I was walking down the Pacific Highway in North Sydney when I took the call. Crying my eyes out, I called my partner, a few close friends, and my sister. "How can this be cancer? But if it is, it must be early." By the time I reached the city I had begun to tell myself "It has to be okay. Don't worry too much." I would get on with my life.

The next week a local surgeon looked at my scans and since it was indeed early, I was triaged and placed at the back of the queue. I understood the pressures on an under resourced regional health system so I contacted my GP to ask whether we could look for a Sydney surgeon who could see me before

Christmas. He got me an appointment with a fantastic surgeon, and at the first meeting, the surgeon and I almost did fist pumps at the results of those first scans. We had caught it so early. My teeny-tiny ballerina boobs were quite muscular and dense so to plan for the lumpectomy surgery, my surgeon suggested a specialist breast MRI to help her see my breast tissue more clearly.

Shortly after the MRI, she called and asked me to come in. The news was not good. I was overwhelmed and the words she used to explain my prognosis triggered emotions and fears that prevented me from absorbing what she told me. She gave me statistics, recurrence, and survival rates but for all that she delivered the information gently and kindly, I could hear only doom and gloom. I could make no sense of it.

The surgeon arranged an appointment with a Breast Cancer Nurse who was meant to help me process and make sense of my diagnosis. All the PR and marketing led me to feel confident—but my crisis only deepened.

When I walked into the small office, the nurse greeted me with a hug but the conversation, like that with the surgeon, did not go well. As she spoke to me, tears welled in her eyes and her voice became hoarse. "Why are you crying?" I asked. The words she chose included "cancer," "stage," "spread," "incurable," "terminal," "survival rates," "chemotherapy," "palliative," and "end of life planning." I won't use these words again in this book because of the damage they can do to a person's identity, sense of self, and capacity to hope for the future. And as I will explain as we make our way through this book, the information provided may not even be accurate. While I appreciate that there is a medical and legal responsibility to cover the full spectrum of possibilities linked to a diagnosis, in terms of the prognosis the reality may be quite different. Later I learned that this nurse was referring to an outdated textbook and didn't seem to be equipped to communicate these messages more effectively.

I knew immediately that the medical professionals had delivered the news that I had cancer in a way that was detrimental. Intuitively, I knew that the narrative and messaging were inconsistent and that I needed to reframe them. To do this, I brought my experience of managing crises in the corporate world into play. I followed my instincts, and they've led me on this path through a life-altering event I at first thought I couldn't endure.

Crisis management strategies can be beneficial in dealing with difficult situations that may arise, whether in your personal or your business life. They are a set of tools you can call on when you feel overwhelmed and need help figuring out what to do next.

A crisis management framework is a structured approach to planning for, responding to, and recovering from a crisis. In terms of your working life, this includes not only policies, procedures, and protocols that can help you prepare for and manage a crisis, but also the roles and responsibilities of other people who are involved. The same broad principles apply in a personal crisis, and in this case the others involved will be your support team.

When you face a crisis, it can feel as though there's no way out. But a systematic approach to dealing with the situation can serve as a roadmap for regaining control.

It's important, too, to be aware that when first faced with a crisis, you may not process information as well as you usually do. Emotions can run high and this, coupled with stress and confusion, can make it difficult to take in and absorb information. Having a crisis management plan in place can provide emotional benefits because the sense of security and peace of mind it provides reduces the anxiety and stress that impede clear thinking. And if the crisis response is well-executed, it can even foster a sense of pride and satisfaction in being part of a team that's making a difference.

Crisis management requires a structured approach and the steps towards feeling more in control in a crisis in your working life are just as effective in the face of a significant personal crisis like a breast cancer diagnosis. In other words, the strategies and tools are universal. In both situations, once the crisis is broken down and understood in its component parts, the steps towards managing it can be tackled one step at a time.

Faced with my crisis, I turned to my craft and training in risk and crisis management. I applied a crisis-management framework and the principles that have been foundational to my work over the last 20 years. Did I know I was doing this at the time? At first, probably not. I swung into action and, almost unconsciously, applied the frameworks I use in my professional work in crisis management to my own situation. I was able to regain control and reach a place of strength and resilience once I had come to terms with uncertainty and recognised the impact of the crisis on my identity.

In the hours after my diagnosis, I was running on adrenaline. I sent text messages to my most trusted friends before contacting my family because I needed to work out what to say to them about what was happening to me and what having this illness meant. I became the CEO role of my own life and knew that my family needed me to speak calmly and confidently, safely. I called my oldest school friend who works in oncology and nursing in New Zealand. We grew up together in the country, where our parents and grandparents lived. We are "cut from the same cloth," as my grandmother would say. My friend understands me and how I tick. I love her like a sister, and I would trust her with my life.

"They have just told me it's serious. It's breast cancer. I've just been delivered this terrible news. Can you please tell me my diagnosis again? Please explain what is happening to me?"

From my training, I knew that once I had a clear understanding of the facts, I would be able to reframe my diagnosis and from there build a strong narrative that would carry me forward.

She explained the difference between breast cancer and other forms of the disease. She explained its treatability. She explained that not only were the data sometimes 10 to 15 years old but that medical advances in breast cancer were occurring so fast that the published data hadn't always caught up. She wanted me to think of it as living with cancer and that it was treatable. Those words changed everything for me. Suddenly there was hope. I wasn't in denial but, rather than fearing there was no way out, I could see a way forward.

Next I had to rally my team because I knew I could not do this alone. I'm fortunate to have relationships with people in corporate and social circles, some of whom could provide me with medical information. I drew on those networks as well as on my friends and family. I explained what was happening to me. I told them my challenges, and people responded with ideas, networks, and skill sets. They carried me through the first emotional stages.

In the initial days following my diagnosis, my primary concern was protecting my family from overwhelming distress. I carefully curated the information I shared with them, providing small updates that satisfied their need to know while shielding them from the full extent of the situation until I had a clearer picture myself. During this time, I found myself leaning heavily on my friends for support, as they became my pillars of strength. They offered unwavering support and understanding, allowing me to express my fears and concerns openly without burdening my family with additional worry. Their strength became my anchor, and together we navigated those early days with a united front, creating a shield of love and support around me and my loved ones.

I also knew that my family would need support, so I quickly put that in place. This was about being open while recognising my own vulnerability and asking for help.

I then needed to build my medical team. I had little confidence in my oncologist early and I knew her communication style would not work well for me. She was focused on data and statistics, and I didn't feel she was looking at me as a whole person. If she had said once more "the data doesn't support this," I don't know what I would've done.

I had to figure out who would provide me with the best care. I had little faith and confidence in the centre I was attending for treatment because of that first diagnosis. If they are delivering cancer diagnoses to women every day, how can they be doing it so badly? Navigating a change of oncologist and surgeon world be difficult. I had to work out where to go and who to ask for help.

After experiencing the overwhelming atmosphere in that initial health space, I realised the importance of assembling a strong and reliable medical team. I began by returning to square one and diligently searching for exceptional general practitioners (GPs). Alongside my primary GP and her team, I sought the assistance of an integrative GP who would serve as my project manager throughout the journey. An integrative GP combines conventional medicine with complementary approaches, providing a holistic perspective on healthcare. With this comprehensive team in place, I felt a sense of relief and stability—a calm port in the storm. They became the trusted individuals with whom I could openly discuss my concerns, make informed decisions, and navigate the complex path ahead. Through this collaborative process, we were able to identify a remarkable oncologist, assemble a dedicated cancer team, and establish a robust support system. It was a journey of discovery, seeking out the right professionals and resources to guide me through the challenges I faced.

When building your medical team, follow your gut. If your gut feels they're not your people, you need to find your people. Breast cancer is treatable, and you will be with these people for a long time—hopefully a very long time.

My next phase was to look for professional support for responding to the emotional aspect of my illness. I was fortunate enough to be supported by a psychologist specialising in health crises. From a safe place, she helped me understand what I was dealing with and talked me through what I was feeling. She also gave me ideas and strategies to manage the inevitable stress. Sometimes when a professional person you trust tells you it's okay to feel as you do, it can make all the difference. She also helped me with how to talk to others. She was my sounding board before I broke the news.

In those first few weeks of the journey, my emotions were everywhere. My strongest feeling was "I don't want this to happen." My body, mind, and soul were fighting this diagnosis so hard. As I broke that down, I could recognise my own fear. I felt afraid. I didn't have enough information to break down that fear and deal with it.

It can feel like you're plugged into a sausage machine when you're diagnosed with breast cancer. Although it is a highly studied and researched form of cancer, sometimes the data means you are dealt with in a pretty linear way. For example, because my psychologist anticipated I would suffer a degree of depression in the face of my diagnosis, she suggested I take pre-emptive antidepressants. Other professionals also warned me of the risk of depression, but I was not depressed in the first few weeks following diagnosis. I did suffer throat-tightening, everything shutting down in waves of anxiety. My understanding, however, is that anxiety exists where there is hope. Depression is more common when there is no hope, when the sufferer can see no way forward. I understand enough to recognise there was hope, but I required help to overcome my fear.

I began a research mission, utilising my medical contacts. I did a lot of reading. This process enabled me to connect with stories of people living well with breast cancer. Yes, it can be a life-limiting disease. Yes, it may reoccur. It may be incurable. However, it is treatable, and there are ways and means of looking after yourself through this process.

With the support of my integrative GP, I came to understand the power of my immune system and the importance of actively taking care of myself to support my body and, hopefully, to slow the replication of cancer cells. To help my body deal with the medication I would need to take, I could take supplements, make changes to my diet, and increase my exercise routine to a point that worked for me. And knowing what I could do to mitigate the crisis I faced meant I regained some control. I had to take the medicine daily, but I could supplement that with things that helped me feel well. And I could go for a spin class or a brisk walk to ensure my medication reached every cell in my body. These things helped my mind to become more robust so that it could support my body's fight. This became a powerful visualisation for me.

Once my recovery regime was clear, I could frame the narrative I would construct to convey to others my journey with breast cancer. Breast cancer, I knew, would affect every aspect of my life, from my private life as a mother to as my public life as a businesswoman—every part of my identity.

Life can move us in unforeseen directions, changing our identity in the process. I saw I would never again be that woman who stood naked in front of a mirror that night in

Melbourne. The sooner I could find the strength to let her go the sooner I would be empowered to become my new self. At the time I didn't understand that what was happening to me was at once a crisis and a gift. Reframing my narrative to take in how I would manage breast cancer and what that meant gave me a great sense of control. It meant that when I articulated my recovery plan to others in my support teams, together we had strength in numbers and a shared narrative. Because we were part of something greater than the cancer, we could work through the crisis together. It also meant that some crippling clichés that have come to be associated with cancer would not influence me as much as they had when I was first diagnosed.

I became frustrated by the stigma attached to a cancer diagnosis. Cancer stigma is a dark cloud that hovers over individuals diagnosed with this devastating disease. It carries the weight of negative attitudes, ignorant beliefs, and hurtful stereotypes. It fuels society's fear and misunderstanding, giving rise to discrimination, isolation, and the spreading of damaging myths. The heavy burden of cancer stigma leaves those affected feeling ashamed, judged, and reluctant to seek the support they desperately need. It casts shadows on their emotional well-being and erects barriers to accessing the care they deserve. Challenging and confronting cancer stigma is essential to illuminate a path of empathy, understanding, and unwavering support for those battling this formidable foe. When I said, "I've got cancer," people didn't always ask, "Oh, what type?" That's an important question to ask because every cancer is different. When I described my cancer, often I could see the person I was speaking to was reflecting on their existing experiences with cancer, many of which, unsurprisingly, were likely to have been quite different from mine.

Each person's journey, including mine, is unique and cannot be compared to others. However, as I shared my experiences with people I encountered, whether they were chance acquaintances or familiar faces, I realised they often interpreted my words through the lens of their preconceived notions. It became necessary for me to look beyond these biases and ensure that those around me understood that my appearance might not reflect my illness. Just because I may appear well doesn't mean I am in remission or free from the daily challenges of living with breast cancer. The goal is to live a fulfilling life despite the obstacles, and shouldn't that be the pursuit we all strive for, regardless of our circumstances?

The power of this reframing on the people around me was remarkable. Like me, they latched onto hope. They saw what they could control, and we were a team. United, we made all the difference to my sense of self and purpose of being.

During a business crisis, the final phase involves reflection, where we carefully contemplate the events that transpired, evaluate successes and failures, identify areas for improvement, and adapt our work practices based on the crisis management experience. However, in a personal crisis, the reflection process is far more extensive. It becomes a daily practice, requiring continuous introspection and flexibility in adjusting our approach. To effectively navigate this introspective journey, I adopt a structured approach to reflection. Breaking down my emotions into manageable components enables me to gain better control over them and derive meaningful insights from the experience.

I will not lie; cancer never leaves my mind. There are moments when I look at my children and think about the grandchildren I may never meet, or that I will miss significant moments in their lives that I had always imagined I would be there for. I will never stop believing I will be there, but I now know nothing is certain. I'm unable to offer you a framework for dealing with these internal conflicts but I don't want to ignore the balance between light and dark because it's the most stunning aspect of life. Joy can't exist without sorrow. A little rain is as essential as sunshine to our wellbeing. In order to experience love, we must accept the possibility of grief. The extent of the emotions aroused is often the measure of the beauty of life.

Dr Toni Lindsay, a clinical psychologist who works primarily in cancer and palliative care in Melbourne, reminds us that certainty is a self-protective myth we use to make sense of a changing world. We accept it blindly until a crisis forces us to recognise that in fact nothing in life is certain. To live our lives in constant fear of, say, being hit by a bus would of course be debilitating but accepting uncertainty gave me a new outlook on how I would live my life after my diagnosis. Life had so much more colour than would have been the case had I not had the terrible news that taught me to live with uncertainty.

I hope that as you read this book you will reflect on my journey. I hope that reading of the devastating despair I've gone through will help you reassess your own situation and so bring more colour to your life too. I hope that reflecting on and applying my professional knowledge and tools—the framework, the roadmap, and the way forward—may reduce the pain you may be going through.

You might think, "How can we apply these strategies and techniques to every crisis? Surely, since every crisis is unique, there'll be some to which they won't apply?" I wasn't sure they would work either, but as I will show, a lot changed when I used these techniques to manage my response to my breast cancer diagnosis.

I will take your hand and guide you as you come to understand why you're experiencing certain feelings and emotions as you face your crisis. Throughout this book, I relate stories of my breast cancer crisis to illustrate how adapting the strategies I use as a crisis PR practitioner actually work in practice. Through my lived experience, you'll be empowered to act in response to your own crisis.

Let's start with a reflection exercise about understanding the impact of a life-altering crisis. Can you recall a time when you experienced a problem or difficult situation in your life?

Think about the emotions you felt, the challenges you faced, and how you responded. Consider how your emotions and thoughts influenced your response to the crisis. Did you feel overwhelmed or uncertain? Did you feel you had control over the situation, or did you feel you were at the mercy of circumstance? Reflect on what you did and what you would like to have done differently to manage your emotions better and respond more effectively. Write your thoughts and reflections in a journal.

In Chapter Nine, we'll reflect more on the value of journaling in reflection and developing your understanding around managing a crisis. By that stage you will know more about the strategies presented in the book and how adopting a systematic approach to a crisis can take you from feeling out of control to feeling secure in the knowledge that you have a roadmap for what lies ahead.

Journaling involves the act of writing down one's thoughts, feelings, and experiences in a personal journal or notebook. It is a form of self-expression and reflection that can be done in various ways, depending on individual preferences and goals. To start journaling, find a quiet and comfortable space where you can focus and let your thoughts flow. You can begin by writing about your day, capturing significant events, emotions, challenges, or any insights gained. Some people prefer a more structured approach, using prompts or specific journaling techniques, while others simply write freely without any constraints.

Journaling serves several purposes. Firstly, it provides a space for self-reflection and self-discovery. By putting thoughts into words, we gain clarity about our emotions, identify patterns, and explore our inner selves. It can also serve as a cathartic release, allowing us to vent our frustrations or anxieties, leading to a sense of emotional relief. Journaling can enhance problem-solving skills, as we analyse situations, brainstorm ideas, and find solutions on paper. Additionally, it becomes a record of our personal growth, capturing memories and insights that we can revisit in the future.

Perhaps you have arrived at this book having already navigated through your personal crisis. If your experience was challenging, revisiting, and reflecting on how you managed it might bring up painful memories. However, it is through this introspective journey that you can gain a deeper understanding of the process you endured. This understanding has the potential to empower you, allowing you to mend any damage caused. Embrace this process and trust in the power of reflection.

The emotional and psychological impacts of a health crisis are complex. But universal principles apply and there is comfort in a shared experience, in hearing another's story and being reminded you are not the only one to have faced such a situation. The crisis may not be your own. You may be part of a support team, and this book includes takeaways supporters, too, may find helpful.

Now reflect on a personal crisis you've faced. It could be a relationship breakup. Having heard my story, how might having this reference point and shared experience have changed your perspective or provided you with the useful tools to manage the situation? It can be hard to reflect on past difficulties. If this is the case, choose one that doesn't trigger deep emotions—receiving a disappointing birthday present, for example. Add your reflection to your journal.

We all need help and guidance in a time of crisis, and I would like to tell you about traps I fell into in the hope you will avoid doing the same. And I want you to know you can change the outcome of a crisis because your knowledge will give you strength and build your confidence as you make your way through the stages of your crisis.

Perhaps your anxiety is such at this stage that you can't imagine how a knowledge of crisis management will help. Understandably, you fear what is ahead, and that fear is paralysing. The sooner you have a plan, a road map, the sooner your anxiety will fade and the sooner you will feel in control. It worked for me. I'd like you to start with self-compassion. Know that whatever you are feeling now is okay. Acknowledge that it's normal to feel overwhelmed in a crisis. Be kind to yourself and know that as you take the journey that is reading and responding to this book, you will achieve an emotional balance that might seem unattainable now. And if at any stage in the process you decide the stress is too much, do as I did when I reached that point and seek professional help.

In this chapter I have described my enormous shock and how it affected me but then led me to develop this book for others. It begins with self-compassion and kindness as it asks you to stop thinking either that the crisis is permanent or that there is nothing you can do. Crisis is painful, but you can and will manage it. Take a deep breath and take comfort. If I could gain control and calm, then you can too. The chapters that follow lay out a process you can follow to manage the crisis; how to trust the process; and how to plan.

## Chapter Two

# The Framework

*"A goal without a plan is just a wish"*

– Antoine de Saint-Expiry

This chapter delves into the foundational systematic understanding of a crisis to help you make sense of why you're feeling the way you do and how best to respond. To help you understand and trust the process, it outlines a management framework, breaking it down into achievable chunks. The rules, stages, and processes form a framework and the better you understand it, the more effectively you will be able to apply it to your crisis.

This chapter breaks down, simply, the crisis management framework I've been using professionally for more than 20 years. I'll show you how to apply this framework to your crisis and how you can tackle a personal crisis using the strategies and ideas businesses use. It will lay the foundation and raise themes I will unpack and discuss in more detail in the chapters that follow. As I suggested in Chapter One, understanding how to approach a crisis systematically will provide you with the security of a roadmap to guide you as you undertake your journey. This is the framework I applied to address the crisis I faced, and I will show you how you can do the same.

One thing I learned early on about having breast cancer is that often the challenge is less the cancer itself than the associated complexities it brings to your life. As I explained in Chapter One, the practical approach I applied to my crisis involved understanding the framework first. When you've been doing something over and over for 20 years, especially in your professional life, patterns become entrenched, and you can't escape them.

The first time I learned this in my crisis was when I was sitting across from my surgeon, listening to her deliver the news. I listened, and for all that I was devastated, I analysed professionally the delivery of her messages as a coping mechanism. In my head, I gave her feedback on her crisis management messaging.

In the first stage of a crisis, you are only sometimes able to reason. Sometimes you lean on instincts like fight or flight: "How am I going to get through this?" "How can I escape this?" You're likely to return to what you know from experience and apply coping skills that are familiar. I am fortunate in that I've picked up many skills through my professional work in crisis management, including putting in place a solid framework from which to proceed. My framework consisted of:

- reframing the diagnosis narrative and seeing clearly what my story looked like.

- forming and rallying my team.
- informing them of the messaging and the shared narrative that we would take forward.
- asking for help.
- being vulnerable.
- being practical.
- sharing examples of what I needed.

I then formed my medical team, which functioned alongside my team of family, friends, and colleagues.

Once these things were in place my support people were able to step in to help me with certain aspects of the crisis. This meant I was less stressed and could find space to think more clearly. I was able to move to a position of control befitting the project manager, the CEO, of my life. Once I was in control, people were able to work with me in a guided, structured way. At that point, I could look back and reflect on what had happened, what needed to be adjusted, and what was yet to be done. My mind was becoming more organised. I had a strategy and I had backing.

Reflection is important. In businesses, we reflect at the end, after the crisis. But as I noted in Chapter One, I've learned that when it comes to a personal crisis, it's important to reflect during the process, too. A systematic approach to reflection gives you a step-by-step process for managing and reframing your crisis.

I'll begin with a definition of crisis, before, with my PR hat on, explaining crisis management. The standard dictionary definition on Google works well for our purposes: a crisis is a situation characterised by intense difficulty or danger, which often involves a critical turning point. For me, the universal application of crisis management strategies and their step-by-step operation, points to how understanding the stages of a crisis prepares you for what to expect and how to respond. Passive emotional responses are reframed to become active strategies. Here I'm applying the framework to a health crisis—my breast cancer crisis. However, as I've already suggested, the application is universal.

A crisis can feel overwhelming and stressful in part because the outcome is so uncertain. You may experience various emotions, including fear, anger, sadness, and confusion. You may feel powerless. The experience depends on the individual and the specific situation, but common symptoms include anxiety, depression, physical stress, difficulty sleeping, difficulty concentrating, and panic attacks. You may feel a strong sense of urgency to act but struggle to decide what action to take. Once you understand the crisis framework, you will know when to act, when to wait, and what to do.

Crisis management, once an academic theory, has now become a widely adopted approach in the PR industry. As I delve into its explanation, it becomes evident that the strategy revolves around a structured process. It begins with defining the crisis and comprehending the full scope of the problem at hand. By breaking it down into stages, this approach effectively counteracts the instinctive fight or flight responses and instead empowers participants to regain control. Anticipating and preparing for what lies ahead becomes key in navigating through the crisis with a proactive stance.

You may be thinking, “But I’m not a PR practitioner. How can I implement this? I’m not sure I’m in a crisis. Perhaps I’m just struggling to cope.” Let me guide you and show you how I responded to my crisis, and you will be able to follow the same steps. The first step is defining your crisis. Reflect on the stages of a crisis you’ve experienced recently and follow the steps to understand how the crisis could be divided into stages. Reflect on whether this understanding might have helped you at any of the stages. While that crisis may have passed, it is useful to reflect on your experience in order to consider strategies you might have used to reframe communications or events damaging to you.

The beautiful thing about the framework is that because it is principles-based it can be applied to any crisis, regardless of its size, scope, or nature. The principles of crisis management—such as assessing risk, communication, and incident management—apply to many crises beyond those that arise in the business community. Depending on the crisis, the principles may vary, but they will often be the same.

This universality has led to the framework's widespread adoption and recognition as a critical aspect of preparedness and response. Worldwide, the crisis management strategies I am speaking of have proved to be essential to preparedness and response from small businesses to multinational corporations, local communities, and national governments.

You may wonder, "How can a one-size-fits-all framework work in every crisis?" Once you understand the framework, you'll feel secure and trust its integrity whether you are in crisis yourself or whether you're a support person or whether you are the person who manages or guides others through it. Outlining the stages and value in understanding is crucial, so you know what to expect and how to respond.

This is a business model, but you will see how readily it translates to a personal one. It follows six specific stages:

- Preparation—creating a crisis management plan, identifying potential crisis scenarios, and developing response protocols.
- Monitoring—monitoring what is happening and staying informed of emerging issues.
- Response—responding to a crisis, including activating our team, releasing official statements to our messaging and social media posts, and taking necessary actions to mitigate the crisis.
- Containment— It is crucial to recognise that many people have limited understanding of cancer, which

can lead to the dissemination of negative or incorrect information. When sharing your breast cancer diagnosis with others, it is essential to be aware that they may project their own perceptions and experiences of cancer onto your situation. As we have highlighted before, cancer types, treatments, sizes, and individual cases can vary significantly. Taking proactive measures to limit the potential damage and control the spread of negative information becomes paramount. By educating others, correcting misconceptions, and advocating for accurate knowledge, we can foster a more informed and supportive environment for those affected by breast cancer.

- Recovery—restoring normal operations, repairing reputation, and implementing the lessons learned to prevent future crises. With breast cancer, this business scenario translates to discovering what your new normal looks like. Life will be different. The affects upon various aspects of your life will be significant, but you will reach a point of life going on.
- Reflection—evaluating the crisis response, identifying areas for improvement, and changing the crisis management plan.

Like other principle-based frameworks, it's important to note that the stages of crisis management may not always follow a strictly linear progression. However, their application remains relevant and valuable regardless of the specific order in which they unfold.

A crisis management framework is a structured approach to planning for, responding to, and recovering from a crisis. It includes all the steps to be taken to prepare for and manage the crisis and to delegate roles and responsibilities to your team. It aims to provide a structured and practical approach to managing the crisis that will ensure you are prepared, responsive, and resilient. I have used this framework daily—from data breaches in big multinational corporations to cyber-attacks, reputation attacks, disasters, and product recalls. In the 20 years I've been using these frameworks, the process and structure rarely, if ever, vary.

Think of a minor crisis you have experience, such as missing a meeting. Using the framework, can you identify the stages of the crisis? Which steps did you, and didn't you, take? Could the framework have helped you? This might be a whole new way of thinking about your life.

Reflecting on your crisis, you might feel overwhelmed emotionally, but it can be a learning experience. There are ways of reframing your feelings in response to a past crisis into the kinds of actions and strategies that will serve you well in the future. When it comes to crisis management, the relationship between emotions and actions is intrinsic. Making plans in advance can have a positive influence on emotions and make hard times easier. Not everyone will experience the same feelings and the severity of crises varies but there is always an opportunity to improve the way we respond. And any improvement will increase your quality of life.

In business, a crisis management plan is essential for several reasons including improved readiness, better decision-making, enhanced reputation, and reduced risk. Regarding the emotional benefits, having a crisis management plan can provide a sense of security and peace of mind. Not only can being prepared reduce anxiety and stress and increase the confidence with which you respond but a well-executed crisis response can give you a sense of pride and satisfaction.

Reframing emerges as the pivotal strategy in your journey towards recovering from the crisis. As I mentioned earlier, my own experience of receiving a diagnosis was fraught with conflicting information. Some of the data presented to me was based on outdated sources, neglecting the transformative progress made in medical advancements over the past eight years. Instead of hearing comforting words like "You can live well with this" or "living with cancer," the initial words that reached my ears were "cancer," "stages," "incurable," "terminal," and various degrees of severity. While these terms are frequently used, they carry a significant weight and shape our perception of the situation. Reframing allows us to challenge and reshape these perceptions, fostering a more empowering and hopeful outlook.

Cancer and the response to it is an individual thing that will vary depending on your type of cancer, its receptiveness to treatment, and how you felt at diagnosis. Were you diagnosed when you were well? Did you already have symptoms? This will vary from person to person, but the labels and words used to communicate the diagnosis can create a trauma from which it is difficult to recover. Reframing allows you to understand your narrative in a way that can be crucial in informing and empowering you and those around you. The process will have an impact on your emotional and, to a degree, your physical who was not only a positive communicator but who was knowledgeable about cancer and delivered diagnoses to people every day. I trusted her. She could provide me with the words, the knowledge, and the positioning I needed to feel a sense of being okay. The diagnosis was still devastating, but I could accept it. I may never accept the prognosis, but after speaking with her, I could feel my anxiety and despair lessen. When I felt afraid, I could turn to these words and remind myself, "This is my story. This is my disease, and this is my type of cancer. These are my circumstances at this point." Once I was strong in that knowledge, I could help and support those around me.

You might be thinking, "My situation is bad. A reframe seems superficial." But your frame of mind and cognitive ability to move forward are essential when you must respond to a crisis. A sense of control and calm will help you to make excellent decisions, rationalise what's happening around you and monitor micro-crises that may come up. You may need, as I did, to change doctors. You may need to change your medication. Being in a place from which you can make sound decisions will empower you.

Let's think of a time when you did a simple reframe. You do it all the time. Perhaps you missed out on a job. Your mind might have jumped to reasons that held you solely responsible: "Was I not good enough? Did I not have enough experience?" But after getting feedback, you might realise that other factors were in play that were not about you. Once you have that information, once you understand the situation, you feel better about it. That, in its simplest form, is a reframe.

We will unpack them further in later chapters, but this chapter teaches you the universal principles and framework you can apply to a crisis. There's no need to feel completely overwhelmed any longer. Use the principles and approach to reframe something that has already happened to be better prepared for the crisis you face now. You can stop wondering whether these techniques apply to you and your situation and start thinking about using these principles now and in the future.

In the next chapter, I'll show you how these principles applied to my crisis and the emotions I experienced. We will think about different frames around your state of mind and your identity, as well as some practical applications and tools that I used as I went from my diagnosis to my ongoing management of my breast cancer.

## Chapter Three

# The Power of Words

***"Be careful with your words, once they are said they can only be forgiven and not forgotten"***

- Unknown

Communication, whether it is helpful or harmful, is particularly powerful in a time of crisis. The need to know what is happening becomes critical because knowledge reduces fear and anxiety. It's essential you know what steps are being taken by your medical team to address the crisis as well as what steps you can take yourself to stay emotionally and physically strong. In the case of a breast cancer diagnosis, for example, clear, accurate, and timely communication promotes not only understanding but also trust, which alleviates anxiety and promotes confidence in your medical and support teams.

In the Introduction, I spoke of my own experience of the impact of outdated negative messages and information communicated to me at the time of my diagnosis. *She Has Breast Cancer* provides you with the skills and strategies so that, should this be your experience, you will be able to reframe those messages in order to address the damage caused. Further, an understanding of how crisis communication works will help you to communicate with your medical and support teams to mobilise them as you journey through your crisis.

Good communication helps manage everyone's expectations by providing precise and consistent information about what is happening now, what is ahead, and what needs to be done. This can help reduce confusion and prevent rumours or any misinformation from spreading. With cancer, this can be important due to the stigma it carries.

In the first few days of my diagnosis, I found it hard to make sense of all the information—much of it contradictory—I was given and to then relay this information to people close to me. I was concerned, for example, about how the words I chose would affect my children and broader family. One way I did this was to ask myself, "What exactly is happening to you?" To answer that question, I had to make sure I had a good grasp of all the information so I could avoid passing on to those around me misunderstandings about my cancer and what my journey would be like for them as well as for me.

I was also concerned about how my news might affect my work and business. Would my clients continue to have confidence in me? Would they, for instance, begin to question my ability and capacity to handle a heavy workload? I also asked whether they would be asking these questions if I had diabetes. The cancer stigma can be heavy.

As emphasised before, the power of language and words cannot be underestimated in shaping our perception of the world. Whether consciously or unconsciously, we often craft messages with the intention to elicit specific emotions in the recipient. Recognising the impact of these messages enables us to identify emotional triggers and assess whether the resulting feelings are appropriate. This awareness becomes instrumental in responding to received messages by reframing negative news, allowing us to view it from a more positive perspective.

For instance, if a message evokes worry or fear, we can shift our focus towards proactive steps to ensure our safety and resilience amidst a barrage of negative and often conflicting information. By reframing the situation, we can concentrate on strategies to remain strong and resilient, safeguarding ourselves from the detrimental effects of such messages.

I will show you the destructive effects on my mental health of the words used to communicate my diagnosis and why, and how, I reframed that narrative so that it supported by wellbeing, and I was empowered.

Understanding how language functions can improve your critical thinking skills and help you evaluate information without being influenced by bias or emotion. In the process, it can help you change how you think and feel not only during a crisis but after it has receded.

At the time of my breast cancer diagnosis, I knew intuitively that the information I was receiving was not only conflicting, but the words and terms chosen were damaging to my mental health. They repeatedly came back to haunt me as I lay awake at 3:00 a.m. However, although words can hurt, they can also nurture and I knew from experience that if I were to reframe the message, it could be empowering rather than damaging.

The story you are told when you are diagnosed, and the story as you reframe it, significantly affect your conscious mind, your subconscious, and your nervous system. In terms of my diagnosis, I was aware from the outset that had I been given more information about survival rates, I would have been better able to take in and respond to what was happening to me.

You might think, "But how can I control what someone tells me and control its impact?" It's true that you cannot control another's narrative even when it's a narrative about you, but you can reflect and gain a greater perspective on what is being said. This means you have the power to reframe it in a way that is more positive, in a way that allows you to see a path through the crisis. Sometimes the news will be bad, but just as there are ways to communicate bad news without damaging the recipient's mental and emotional state, there are ways the recipient can receive and process that news. The recipient need not be passive.

Reflect on a time when someone gave you bad news. What was the message? Who delivered it and how? How did you feel? Could there have been a different way of communicating the news, and of receiving it? It may be painful to revisit this event but think of it as an opportunity to reframe it so that it no longer causes unnecessary suffering. The knowledge you will gain will help you to both communicate bad news and to receive and reframe it in future.

Understanding the importance of good communication from your medical professionals will empower you to demand it. Finding a doctor who communicates and instils trust is a crucial step in ensuring you receive the treatment you need.

If I had the opportunity to educate medical workers about communicating a diagnosis, my advice would be that they:

- Choose a private place and ensure everyone is comfortable before a diagnosis is broached.
- Avoid medical jargon. In the case of a cancer diagnosis, avoid specific terms such as terminal or aggressive that may or may not be associated with the patient's journey.
- Express empathy and compassion for the patient and their family; acknowledging their feelings and concerns.
- Provide clear, accurate and comprehensive information, including the diagnosis, prognosis, and treatment options.
- Address the positive as well as the negative aspects of the diagnosis. For example, breast cancers are often treatable, and medical advances are occurring all the time. This information could have enabled me respond more actively to my diagnosis from the outset.

- Encourage the patient to ask questions, and provide them with clear, honest answers.
- Provide guidance in the knowledge that at this early stage they may not know what questions to ask.
- Allow time for the patient to process the information you have communicated.
- Offer links to resources such as counselling or breast cancer support groups you know to be of the highest standard.
- Schedule a follow-up appointment to check in on the patient and answer questions that may have arisen.

So good channels of communication must be put in place at the outset. Don't be afraid to ask, "How can I best communicate with you if I have questions?" In the couple of days following my diagnosis, I had a lot of questions, and my surgeon was happy for me to email them.

As I have intimated, the conversation around my diagnosis was clumsy and damaging. Not only was the future they painted one of unrelieved doom and gloom, but the information was unclear and at times contradictory. Practitioners used common cancer terms without distinguishing between breast and other cancers, and, because of a mix-up in patient records, a nurse gave me an incorrect diagnosis. I thought, "Goodness if they're doing this a couple of times a day every day, why are they getting it so wrong? If experts in the field are unable to wade through the information, how will I manage?" I lost faith in this medical team and the relationship could not be repaired.

You might think, "But aren't all medical professionals taught doctor-patient communication?" Not necessarily. According to my research, communication is not always considered a fundamental skill, and practitioners will often study it after completing their core education. It's viewed as something along the lines of professional development and so it's a choice a practitioner might or might not take up

As I have begun to suggest, with even a basic understanding of crisis communication, you can reset or reframe damaging conversations; you can reframe a story so that it better assists you in your journey. This reframing might involve seeking out support networks that will enable you to better understand your situation and counter misinformation.

Talking to someone you trust, such as a friend or family member, can help reduce the negative emotions that block your active processing of the news. More formal support from mental health professionals, such as a therapist or counsellor, can help you work through the messaging to create a storyline that will support your physical and mental health.

Taking care of yourself through exercise, meditation, or just making time for yourself can also help reduce stress and promote a more positive outlook. In times of crisis, it's helpful to focus on those aspects of your life you can control, such as the promotion of your physical and mental wellbeing, rather than dwelling solely on your diagnosis. Agency is empowering.

I undertook one of the most powerful reframes of my diagnosis with the help of my clinical psychologist. She asked me to think of my illness not as breast cancer but as a life-impacting chronic illness that would need treatment forever. Yes, it could be a life-limiting illness, but she reminded me that medical advances meant new treatments were becoming available all the time. The impact on my mental health was significant. That hope enabled me to focus on the moment and to feel positive about tomorrow, and my hope gave strength to those supporting me. Knowledge is power, and the more you know and understand, the better you will be able to reimagine a path forward.

Reframing is a powerful learned skill—it is difficult and takes practice, but you can master it, one step at a time.

As I have suggested, the culture of medicine has always emphasised technical proficiency and scientific knowledge above soft skills like doctor-patient communication. However,, the research shows a clear relationship between a patient's emotional and psychological response on receiving a traumatic diagnosis and their subsequent wellbeing. Those who experience distress and anxiety are more likely to lack confidence in their subsequent medical treatment and to suffer adverse outcomes such as depression and reduced quality of life. On the other hand, patients who are able to manage the emotions they feel on diagnosis and are confident about their medical treatment, are more likely to experience better outcomes.

Several factors beyond communication can influence the response to a diagnosis, including the type and severity of the disease, overall mental and emotional circumstances, personal coping style, and the support systems available.

Once I found a medical team I could communicate with, we were able to develop a relationship based on trust. My perspective shifted because I knew that even if the worst happened, I could depend on my team. For all that I would continue to be actively engaged in my treatment, I could, to a degree, trust my team to make decisions about me or for me. I trusted that I was in expert hands and that I'd be called on when we needed to make decisions together but that I could set my medical care to one side as I got on with my life. For me, it was and is a positive relationship.

You may ask yourself, "But what if my doctor is a poor communicator? I can't change that, can I?" Perhaps not, but since you will have an ongoing relationship with this professional, it may be that one of the decisions you will make as you take an active role in your future wellbeing will be to find a doctor who *is* a good communicator.

When it comes to communication at the time of a medical diagnosis, I get it. We see doctors as experts, authorities in a rarefied field, so we not only tend to defer to their knowledge, but we tend to lower our expectations of their capacities in areas that are not strictly defined as medical. But knowing how important good communication is for your mental and physical health outcomes, consider how poor communication might affect your response to treatment.

Let's return to the myth of certainty and the concept of uncertainty. It took me some time to understand the concept, and why we form expectations around the illusion of certainty, but understanding it was a vital step forward in reframing my crisis. We humans crave stability and predictability, which is to say we crave certainty. It gives us a comforting sense of security and control in the face of a patently unpredictable and chaotic world. We choose to rely on experiences and patterns to make assumptions about the future, and we choose to believe that specific outcomes are inevitable when the reality is that life is inherently unpredictable and the unexpected can occur at any time.

In a crisis, grief for the loss of certainty may manifest itself in anxiety, stress, and confusion all which compound feelings of helplessness and vulnerability and make it difficult to make sound decisions.

In reality, none of us can face the future with certainty. We just don't recognise that certainty is a myth. People said to me during my crisis, "Oh my goodness, are you making plans? What are you going to do?" My response was, "What plans are you making?" Yes, I have more information about my illness, and this means I have plans for managing it in the future. But what about the person hit by a bus this morning? What about the person savaged by a shark while on holiday? Had they made plans for such a crisis? Probably not, because they, like me, were probably attached to the myth of certainty and repressed the reality that uncertainty is a normal part of life.

Grieving the loss of certainty is a natural response to a crisis but we can learn to adapt to change. People around you may struggle with this in part because they project their uncertainty of their own future on you. It's the old story—if it's not you, it's me. You may face situations in which you feel isolated and vulnerable—a friend might cross the street to avoid talking to you because of the uncomfortable feelings your situation brings up for them. You may be a reminder or trigger for their subconscious awareness of the uncertainty of their own future.

Letting go of certainty allows you to be more open-minded, flexible, and able to adapt to new experiences and ideas. Anxiety and stress are reduced as soon as it's no long necessary to control the fear of the unknown. By embracing uncertainty, you may discover new opportunities and possibilities previously overlooked. You will be able to live life in colour and in the moment. Each of us is dying, so why don't we allow our lives to reflect the value of every day in the face of uncertainty?

A dear family friend who is a war veteran spoke to me about these months after my diagnosis. He recognised that I was living life on the edge and that I was feeling the exhilaration, the joy in that. He likened it to waking up every day on the battlefield, knowing that today could be your last, not knowing whether you would come home.-"It's no different for you," he said. Humans are unique in compartmentalising aspects of their lives and getting on with the day-to-day despite everything. There is a feeling of exhilaration when you reach the point you've accepted uncertainty. You start living in a place of gratitude and see life in colour, bright colour.

What does this have to do with communication? Everything. It's often the concepts that are first communicated to us that we hold on to when we receive a diagnosis and letting go of it can help you. Communication during a crisis is crucial and knowing how messages affect you can help manage emotional distress. This awareness can also help you communicate effectively as your crisis progresses. Remember that if your diagnosis was communicated badly, or if you have had a bad interaction with a doctor, think about the value of a strong relationship with your medical team. Focus on communication because it's one thing that you can control.

Pause for a moment to contemplate the nature of your connection with your medical team and the profound impact it may have on you. This aspect might hold more significance than you realise, shaping various aspects of your well-being and overall experience.

In the next chapter, we will look at the health system—and how you can fight to ensure it works for you, so you don't have to fight for your life.

# Chapter Four
# Understanding the Business of Health

*"Man, the living creature, the creating individual, is always more important than any established style or system"*

- Bruce Lee

Since being diagnosed with breast cancer I have felt increasing anger and resentment towards much of the PR surrounding aspects of treatment and support. If I had believed all the PR from the pink charities, I would have expected a plush red carpet to have been rolled out leading me to an array of support and services. It was not the case either for me or for many women I have spoken to.

Let's start with the fallacy of early detection. Early detection strategies, such as mammography screening, have limitations and are not fool proof. Mammography can miss up to 20% of breast cancers, particularly in women with dense breast tissue. At the same time, mammography can detect small tumours that might not have progressed to become clinically significant or life-threatening, leading to overdiagnosis and overtreatment.

Another factor is that the benefits of early detection may vary depending on the woman's age and individual risk factors. For example, younger women have denser breast tissue, which can make detecting breast cancers with mammography challenging.

Not only can these limitations and variations in the effectiveness of early detection strategies impact on diagnoses for younger women being screened for breast cancer but negative mammogram results can lead to a false sense of security resulting in delayed diagnosis and delayed treatment.

Further, the detection of non-life-threatening tumours can lead to overtreatment, causing unnecessary anxiety and physical harm to patients.

But of course, early detection remains a critical component of breast cancer screening, and mammography is still the most effective tool for detecting early-stage breast cancer in women over 50. However, what many of us don't know is that for younger women alternative screening strategies, such as MRI or ultrasound, may be more appropriate. For this reason, women should consult their healthcare provider to determine the best screening approach based on their individual risk factors.

Again, it's about knowledge and making informed decisions. A study published in the *Australian Health Review* 2016, found that patients who were more knowledgeable about the healthcare system were more likely to engage in shared decision-making with their providers and this led to more positive healthcare experiences.

Once you understand "the business of health" and how it works you will be able to navigate what can be a complex, even convoluted, system to achieve the best outcomes. What are the roles of healthcare providers, insurance companies and government agencies? This knowledge will, for example, help you to choose a healthcare provider that will provide the best care and, should it be necessary, help you to negotiate better coverage.

Understanding how different aspects of the system are funded allows you to see not only why some services are easily accessed and some are not but also how best to advocate for yourself to ensure you get the care you need. Because you know how the system works, you will be able to challenge insurance denials, negotiate medical bills, and even identify ways of accessing financial help through charities. Understanding the business of health has helped me to make better decisions.

In this chapter, we'll look at some of the frailties of the breast cancer industry and the challenges patients face. While Australia has a relatively high level of government spending on healthcare, there are concerns about the sustainability of the current funding model in the face of growing demand across all sectors of the system. Although Medicare is a universal healthcare system, funding cuts have meant those living in rural or remote areas have for some time found it difficult to access the services they need, and those in urban areas have begun to experience similar difficulties. As healthcare costs, private and public, have increased, funding has not kept up. There are many reasons for this. Our ageing population is growing rapidly. Mental health is a growing issue, with high rates of anxiety and depression reported, particularly among young people. The incidence of chronic diseases is increasing. Advances in medical technology are beneficial but they are expensive. All these issues are exacerbated by shortages of trained healthcare professionals and hospital beds. Waiting times for appointments as well as treatment are coupled with compromised standards of care as healthcare workers and facilities like hospitals and care facilities are stretched to breaking point.

Understanding how these challenges are affecting the services you will need to access will help you assess whether and where you will need to push to get the care you require. Knowing which sectors are under pressure, and what those pressures are, will help you and your medical team to keep your treatment on track.

You may be thinking, "Why wouldn't I just trust the system?" While the quality of the Australian healthcare system is the envy of many similar countries, I would reiterate how important it is that you participate in your health-care program. This involves asking questions, understanding your diagnosis and treatment options, and getting a second opinion—or even a new team—when necessary. Being an active participant and advocate for your own healthcare means you will be active in accessing the best possible care, and the best possible outcome, the system can deliver.

Reflect on your last illness or even your current one. If you have faced, or are facing breast cancer, have particular aspects of your illness or your treatment created challenges for you? Do you wish you had had more advocacy and support? There are pros and cons for our healthcare system of health and having a knowledgeable, balanced view will help you understand challenges instead of allowing them to negatively influence your journey. At the same time, despite the best intentions of trained and experienced healthcare professionals, and despite electronic medical records and medical management systems, mistakes can still occur and there is no doubt errors in diagnosis, medication, and treatment have serious consequences.

Healthcare in Australia is becoming increasingly commercialised, with private healthcare providers and pharmaceutical companies having more influence on policy and funding decisions than is healthy. This can lead to conflicts of interest and prioritisation of profits over patient care.

A good friend and wise woman recently pointed out to me that it is called a medical "practice" for a reason. In the context of medicine, the term "practice" refers to the habitual work of healthcare, but it also refers to the professions' constant evolution that is a result of new research, new technologies, and new understandings of the human body. Doctors, like other healthcare providers, rely on existing learning and experience, but at the same time they are always learning and improving their skills, and each patient presents a unique challenge that requires a tailored approach. We might then recognise medicine not as a fixed science, but rather as an ongoing process of learning and adaptation. Healthcare providers are always "practising" and refining their skills and knowledge. To recognise that medicine as a practice is to remind ourselves of the ever-evolving nature of the field and the lack of complete knowledge or certainty in areas, such as cancer treatment. Cancer is a complex disease. Increasingly it is recognised that there is no "one size fits all" approach to its treatment, and that doctors must constantly adapt their knowledge and techniques to best serve each individual patient and their unique experience of the disease. This in turn reminds us of the importance of personalised care and the need for patients to be actively involved in their treatment decisions

And this brings us to precision medicine. Precision medicine is is a new approach that uses information about your genes and their associated proteins to prevent, diagnose, or treat a disease. The National Cancer Institute explains that "precision medicine uses specific information about a person's tumour to help make a diagnosis, plan treatment, find out how well treatment is working, or make a prognosis."

How does it differ from current treatments? Under current treatment plans, if there is a 75% chance that treatment A will work, then you'll get treatment A. It's a blind choice based on a protocol and does not take account of the individuality of cancer. Sometimes, it can be five full lines of treatment until they get the right one—and often that is too late. We need to fight for the right drug first, every time. While this may be expensive, and it will require a wholesale change from education through to economics and practice, there needs to be more funding going to scientific partners who make this happen.

When I learned about precision medicine, choosing it seemed like a straightforward decision. Wouldn't you just test the patient to discover the best treatment for them? When I asked my oncologist about this, she replied that the preference is to wait until other treatments are failing because the test is expensive. "So, you wait until it's too late?" I asked. My question was met with silence. As patients we need to empower ourselves to address negative experiences like this. Asking questions and insisting on answers is just one of the effective strategies we can each develop as we address your own crisis. Understanding who the different players and resources are can also help you develop a strategy that considers the different interests and priorities. You might be thinking that this sounds too hard to navigate by yourself and yes, sometimes you'll need to pull in extra support, but as I've already suggested, in a crisis preparedness for what is ahead is a strategy.

Reflect on your last experience in a hospital. Were you aware you were observing a system under pressure? If not, would this awareness have helped you to get the system working for you?

To receive optimal care, it is crucial that you have a clear understanding of your healthcare requirements, as well as those of your family. This involves staying informed about your medical history, including any chronic conditions and specific needs you may have. By being well-versed in your healthcare needs, you can effectively communicate with healthcare providers, such as Medicare, private health insurance companies, and community health services. Having knowledge about the services and benefits offered by each entity empowers you to make informed decisions and choose the most suitable options available. This is yet another essential aspect of taking an active role in managing your healthcare.

How can you best support your body while it's going through treatment? Are there, for example, dietary supplements you could take to help your body deal with the effects of pharmaceutical medications? You should be able to ask your medical team questions like this. These are good questions to ask and if you're not happy with the care, you're receiving or you feel that you're not being heard, it's important to advocate for yourself. This includes speaking up and expressing your concerns, seeking second opinions, or making complaints.

I wish I had spoken up for myself sooner about being screened for breast cancer. I asked several medical professionals at the time of my mother's diagnosis during the COVID-19 pandemic and the answer was, "You don't need to be tested. You're too young, you're not high risk. You can't feel anything, so why would we test you?" At the time the medical system as a whole was under pressure because of the pandemic. Services were shutting down and indeed BreastScreen NSW was closed for a period. But if I had advocated for myself earlier and insisted on being tested, the entire course of my journey might have been different. While it is true that women under 50 can develop breast cancer, it is important to note that the eligibility criteria for mammogram appointments at BreastScreen may differ. Due to the consideration of risk factors and effectiveness, it may be more challenging for women under 50 to secure an appointment. BreastScreen, in line with its guidelines, primarily focuses on providing mammograms for women aged 50 to 74, as evidence suggests that this age group benefits the most from regular screening. However, it is advisable for women of all ages to consult with their healthcare provider regarding breast health and appropriate screening options based on their individual circumstances.

Yet in all the waiting rooms in the breast care centres I attended during my diagnosis, the women were all my age or younger. I imagine they have stories like mine. Breast cancer is a significant health issue in Australia and the breast cancer industry faces a range of challenges. Although there's a national breast screening program in Australia, some of us face barriers, as I did, when it comes to access.

There is also a need for increased participation in breast cancer clinical trials in Australia. This is important for patients with aggressive or advanced breast cancer who may have limited treatment options. It is important, too, for those population groups in Australia that experience higher rates of breast cancer and poorer outcomes. These include First Nations women, women from lower socioeconomic backgrounds, and women from diverse backgrounds. Breast cancer survivors may experience ongoing physical, emotional, and psychological challenges outside of their illness and there is a need for more support services and resources to help survivors manage the long-term effects of a disease.

Despite Medicare, the cost of breast cancer treatment can be a barrier to accessing care for some Australians, particularly those without health insurance. There are many breast cancer charities in Australia and it's an industry that raises millions of dollars each year, but it has faced criticism in recent years regarding the allocation of funds and their impact on women with breast cancer. A fundamental problem is a lack of coordination and collaboration among organisations leading to duplication.

Further, some organizations have been accused of prioritising funding for popular or "sexy" initiatives, such as awareness campaigns or fundraising events, over research that might lead to significant breakthroughs in breast cancer prevention and treatment.

Some critics have argued that the breast cancer industry has become commercialised, with companies and organisations using the international pink ribbon symbol to sell products and services without contributing significantly to the cause.

Pink has always been my favourite colour, a hue I cherished dearly. However, everything changed after my diagnosis. The clichéd association that pink carried began to repel me. Instead of concealing my affection for this colour, I boldly embraced it. I refuse to let myself be defined by these stereotypes. I am determined to reclaim my favourite colour, to celebrate it without restraint. These clichés, after all, are being exploited for monetary gain.

We need to demand transparency and accountability from the charitable industry to allocate funds to where women need it most. Organisations must disclose their financial information and how they allocate their funds, and there must be an emphasis on investing in research that will have the greatest impact on improving breast cancer outcomes. Transparency would enable donors to do their research and support organisations that have a proven track record of supporting breast cancer patients and research.

Understanding the challenges of the breast cancer industry may help you when you encounter barriers on your own journey. Again, I would encourage you to empower yourself by doing your own research so you can formulate the questions you need to ask before you face what you are dealing with. When I was diagnosed, I felt overwhelmed and so I researched the challenges of the breast cancer industry, knowing this would empower me to ask the questions I needed answered. Even on websites that were recommended as safe and informative, I encountered unhelpful and conflicting messages. I noticed a significant focus of PR and marketing efforts around breast cancer targeting an older demographic, which made it challenging for me as a younger individual to relate to the information provided.

The perception of breast cancer is that it is an over-fifties cancer and here I was at 42, facing the same battle as that faced by older women but with quite different challenges. It was very hard to join the dots and map the services I could, as a younger woman, access.

Reflect on the extent to which you have benefited from the services on offer. What could have helped you better access help and support? If you are one of those who doesn't enjoy taking part in cancer services because of cancer's associations, I would recommend you look for a generalist service. Knowing how the health system functions as a business and operates as an ecosystem can assist you to navigate it and find strategies that will allow you to achieve your best health outcomes. Stop trusting the system. It may be better to put your energy into fighting a broken system than ending up having to fight for your life because the system failed you. You are the patient, and the health system is there for you. Don't feel that you are there for it. Be assertive and put yourself first.

In the next chapter, we will discuss what I term the identity-theft aspect of cancer. Words can become labels, and those labels can become your identity. The impact of this in a health crisis is significant and can undermines the confidence that is so important to achieving the best outcome. Once you understand the process, you can transform and rebuild your mindset. You won't be the same person, but your rebuild can turn into an empowering and positive experience.

## Chapter Five

# Labels and Identity

*"A girl should be two things: who and what she wants."*

— **Coco Chanel**

Words possess a profound ability to shape our very essence, forming the labels that define our identity. In the midst of a health crisis, the weight of negative labels can erode the self-assurance vital to our well-being. You might find yourself burdened by the label of a mere patient, a cancer patient, or worse, a victim. Yet, within this journey, there exists a transformative process, a journey of rebirth. Understanding this metamorphosis becomes a beacon of hope, empowering us to rebuild our shattered selves. While we may emerge forever changed, the strategies and tools shared within these pages hold the power to ignite an ember of strength, guiding us towards an empowering renaissance.

Words possess the remarkable power to define and confine, like sticky glue that clings relentlessly. As I will explore, these labels become etched into our very essence, shaping our identity. Alas, when negativity seeps into these labels, their effects can be devastating. Cancer, too, falls victim to this pattern, burdened by connotations and labels that inflict wounds. They chip away at our confidence and self-worth, leaving us feeling inadequate and disconnected, while a crumbling self-assurance can sow seeds of ill health.

But there is hope. Even though labels can become part of your identity, that identity isn't set in stone. With the right tools and a strong enough mindset, you can reject the label and turn your experience into something positive and empowering. I won't lie—it's not going to be easy, but it is possible. In the end, you might not be the same person you were before, but that's okay. You'll be stronger and more resilient. Let's throw off those labels and rebuild ourselves!

Identity is all about who you are and what makes you unique. It's what sets you apart from everyone else in the world. A crisis can disrupt your normal routine and the ensuing uncertainty and chaos can leave you feeling lost and disoriented. You may feel as though you no longer know who you are or what your purpose might be. If you experience a traumatic event during a crisis, it can have a lasting impact on your sense of self. You may feel your world has been turned upside down and you are struggling to find your footing. That happened to me. Not only did other people give up on me, but I gave up on myself for a time. I was constantly thinking of what I was losing, and it took me almost three months to see what I was gaining.

Your identity shapes your sense of self. It's what gives you a sense of belonging and helps you understand your place in the world. When you know who you are, you become more confident, and this means you are in a position to make better decisions for yourself. And your identity is what connects you to other people. It's what helps you form relationships and build community. For example, identifying with others going through experiences like yours can make you feel less alone and more supported. But here's the thing: your identity is unique. Nobody else has quite the same experiences or background as you do. That's why it's so important to embrace your identity and own it. When you do that, you show the world you're proud of who you are. That's a powerful thing, and it can have a significant impact upon those around you.

A crisis can shake that sense of identity, so don't hesitate to seek support from loved ones or professionals as you rebuild.

In this chapter, I'm going to talk through some of the softer skills and concepts you can call on—the thought-provoking stuff that will help you kick along and will inspire your reframe process.

As I have begun to suggest, your identity, how you see yourself and how others perceive you, is defined not only by the way you act in the world but also by others' perception of you and the words used about you. These words can have a significant impact on how you see yourself and how others see you. These perceptions shape your self-esteem and confidence and thus your identity. Negative language—such as unkind, ugly, or stupid—can cause you to feel you have no value. On the other hand, positive language—such as kind, intelligent, or beautiful—can boost your self-esteem and allow you to feel good about yourself. The words used about you can influence how others perceive you, too. If someone speaks positively about you, others are more likely to see you in a positive light.

Words used to describe your health, wellbeing, and physical capacities, particularly at the time of a cancer crisis, have a similar effect. They conjure up perceptions or emotions and have extraordinary suggestive powers over your body and how it's feeling.

One of the reasons I started this book's title with "She" came from when I was lying on a bed waiting for a liver biopsy. I was slightly sedated. People were walking around me, holding clipboards, computers, and scans. They kept referring to me in the third person. "She needs this test." "She needs a Medicare card." They weren't talking to me; they were talking about me. I listened to some of the other words they were using and started to pay attention to how it was making my physical body and my heart feel about myself. It was disturbing.

Since the language used to describe you can shape how you see yourself and how others see you, and since that process can have a significant impact not just on your identity and self-esteem but on your overall health, it's essential you are mindful of just what words are used and the effects they are having.

When I was first diagnosed, I remember sitting in the surgeon's office. Reflecting on it now, the atmosphere was sombre. From the moment I entered the room, her face said it all. It reflected her view of my diagnosis and its prognosis. It was negative, dark, and gloomy. She didn't qualify the statistics she was giving me. She didn't tell me about the advances in treatments. In other words, she didn't give me information that would have allowed me to take in what the diagnosis would mean for me.

When I connected with a second medical team, the contrast could not have been greater. They delivered their diagnosis in a way that allowed me to process what I needed to know. They talked about my disease but also about longevity. They explained they were in control and were focused on giving me the best health and best life possible. It was up to me to go out and live it. They talked about advances in the treatment of breast cancer and how they would impact my treatment. It was individualised. It was about me. They were looking at me, not "she."

My new team allowed me to see the positives and I felt confident because they were confident in their knowledge, research, and treatments. My oncologist asked me a lot of questions about my life and when I told her that I'd scaled back work, she asked "Why? I'm looking after your health and giving you the best life, you can, so go and live it." The impact on my physical being, my heart, and my confidence was palpable. The change came down to two types of communication style.

Only 60 days since my first diagnosis, I was the same patient and nothing had changed in my records, yet the change to how I felt about my situation was incredible.

I remember the hours and the night that followed from the initial diagnosis. As I lay awake in a hotel room, it became clear to me that my thoughts were being shaped by the words used to deliver my diagnosis. I couldn't get them out of my head. My experience reminded me of my work in crisis management and how we teach businesspeople how crucial good communication is in the first 24 hours of a crisis. You need to get it right.

I remember walking out of the hospital after the first meeting with my new team. I walked back into life. I did not look back. I set aside my diagnosis as I got on with my day. At home later that night, I lay in bed and reflected on the day and particularly about the words that were used to explain what was happening to me. This time my thoughts were positive. There was hope. My cancer was treatable. The people who were going to treat me knew what they were doing. They were going to help me live.

You might be thinking, "But shouldn't we just be focused on the technical side of our care?" Of course, the technical side is important. However, when you're experiencing a long-term illness, over time communication will have an impact on your physical health. Look at the impact on me of two modes of delivering my diagnosis.

"Sticks and stones may break my bones, but words can never hurt me." From my experience, the latter part of the old proverb is not true; in fact, it's a damaging form of denial. As I have already stated, how people speak about you and how they speak to you can affect your self-perception positively or negatively, and the effect is even more immediate in a time of crisis. You need to recognise when words are indeed hurting you.

Think of the last time you lay awake at 3.00 am. What were the thoughts that were keeping you from sleep? What were the words that gave rise to those thoughts? They were obviously powerful. What difference might different words have made?

There is a laziness in language in the medical industry and because communication is not valued enough, the language and modes of communication used are not updated or refined as rapidly as research and technology are changing medical practice. A perfect example of this is the different narratives or stories used around breast cancer. On the one hand, the reality of cancer can be difficult and scary to face, especially when you consider statistics around survival rates. But on the other, breast cancer treatment has come a long way and progress is being made every day.

The second narrative distinguishes between breast cancer and other types of cancer in that not only is breast cancer more often treatable but there are many treatment options. The research shows that mental health and a positive mindset are helpful in managing treatment, side effects and recovery.

Communicating this to patients in a way that is both clear and hopeful is a challenge to which the breast cancer industry too often doesn't rise. Collectively, the industry, which Breast Cancer Action defines as the agencies, organisations and corporations that protect and fail to protect our health, could better work together to communicate the realities and the possibilities of breast cancer treatment. Medical practitioners could emphasise the progress that has been made and the many treatment options available while still being honest about the challenges. They could provide patients with the resources and support they need to manage the emotional and psychological aspects of breast cancer treatment. These resources might include access to counselling or support groups, as well as educational materials designed to help patients understand their diagnosis and treatment options.

Women with breast cancer can be empowered and hopeful in the face of their diagnosis. Focusing on better communication support will help to improve the overall quality, care, and outcomes for women with the disease and this will affect families, communities, and our overall society. According to the latest statistics from the Australian Institute of Health and Welfare, an estimated 55 women are diagnosed with breast cancer every day in Australia. The kind of poor communication I experienced can affect every one of those women as they face a serious disease that will have a significant impact their physical and emotional wellbeing. Fifty-five women every day; over 20,000 women every year. Imagine the impact poor communication of a diagnosis has not just on each of these women but on society. Women are our mothers, caregivers, and an integral part of our societal life.

You might ask, as I did after that first diagnosis, "Why do they seem to know so little or have a way of managing something they work with every day?" I asked that question again after the second diagnosis. My case is a prime example that there is not a standardised approach. Think about your own experience of diagnosis. How did you, or the person you supported, handle the news? It may be painful to reflect, but perhaps looking at it from the perspective of how far you have come since your diagnosis will lead to empowerment.

It is important for patients to recognise whether their diagnosis was delivered well or poorly because of its potentially lasting emotional and physical effects. If a diagnosis is communicated poorly, you may feel confused and overwhelmed. You may feel your concerns and questions haven't been, and won't be, taken seriously or that your healthcare provider doesn't care about you as an individual. This can block future communication. It's important to know what steps you can take to deal with what can be a traumatic experience. This might mean talking to a therapist or finding a new healthcare provider with whom you feel more comfortable.

Knowing your diagnosis was delivered poorly and the implications of that for your health can also enable you to speak up and make positive changes in the healthcare system itself. By sharing experiences, as I am, you can raise awareness about the importance of clear and caring communication in healthcare. This can improve the way healthcare providers talk to patients and make sure everyone gets the best care possible.

My gut feeling that my treatment during the time of my diagnosis wasn't right was validated by my experience with the second team. The damage not only to my mental health but to that of those around me was unnecessary and it hurt. But I did learn how to communicate what I needed, and I tried a few cancer care centres, rather as I used to try new shoes, until I found my place. From the receptionist to the consultant specialist, their communication, culture, and approach was strong, supportive, and consistent. At the first appointment I learned more about my illness than I had in the previous two months, and our relationship is as close to perfect as you can get in this business.

I felt further vindicated in my decision to seek out the care I needed when they told me that, given my long-term prognosis and the fact that my cancer is slow growing, they would help me access treatment as close to precision medicine as the system allowed. Of course, it's still a scary illness and things could change, but the lesson I learned over the first months following my diagnosis was to put myself and my care first.

Your response might be "But I'm just one person. How can I advocate for myself?" My answer is, quite simply, the one this book has focused on: "You have to take responsibility for your care."

When you reflect on the first few months of your diagnosis or that of your loved one, do you recognise a gap between what you had imagined you would find, based on what is projected by the breast cancer industry, and what you in fact experienced? When I walked into the breast cancer world, I imagined I would be supported. Perhaps you were as surprised by the reality as I was.

At first you may not have the confidence to speak up. Start small as you grow your strength. You might begin with something as simple as not wanting to be weighed in the public waiting room. Or maybe you want to attend a different blood test provider because their location is more convenient for you. It's important that you start to build that speaking-up muscle because you're going to be using it often.

I actively pushed for good communication with the forward-thinking medical team I had chosen to help guide me, because not knowing what to expect can result in uncertainty and anxiety. Of course, healthcare professionals will not always be able to predict the outcome of cancer treatment despite the new technologies that are changing the landscape of cancer treatment and improving outcomes, including targeted therapies, immunotherapies, and precision medicine that are allowing doctors to better understand the genetic makeup of cancer cells and to develop more personalised treatment plans based on an individual's unique needs. Advances in imaging and diagnostic tools are enabling earlier detection and more accurate staging of cancers. As a result, patients are experiencing improved outcomes and better quality of life, with some even achieving complete remission. While there is still much work to be done in the fight against cancer, these new technologies are providing hope for the future and a brighter outlook for cancer patients and their families. The right specialists can offer support, hope, and the latest information on treatment options and potential outcomes. By working together, my healthcare professionals and I cultivated the kinds of positivity and forward thinking that gave me the confidence that empowered me in my journey.

Communication is the process of exchanging information, ideas, and thoughts between individuals or groups. It's a skill we use every day to interact with others as we make sense of the world around us. You need to become a Master of Communication. It's a learned skill, and by mastering it you can control, to some extent, your sphere of influence and achieve the outcomes you desire. This applies as much to your health as to any other sphere. Effective communication will foster strong relationship with your medical team and your support team.

To become a Master of Communication, you will need to develop your listening skills, be aware of your body language, choose your words carefully, and be open to the needs and perspectives of your audience.

Communicating my story was something I worked on with the help of my psychologist. I wanted to be sure I communicated factual information that reflected my approach to responding to my diagnosis. It was also important to me that my family and friends were able to communicate the same messages to others as they needed to. Cancer carries an extraordinary stigma, and I wanted to break that down as much as I could for me and those around me.

To communicate more widely what was happening to me, I created a social media post. I put a great deal of care into ensuring it was not only an accurate account of what I was going through that would not only circumvent gossip but also assist those around me to support me in my approach:

> *So, we call this Living with a Treatable Cancer. The experts like it to be framed as a chronic, life-threatening, life-limiting illness that needs treatment for longevity. I want to give you all the information because the stuff out there on the old World Wide Web is terribly outdated, some of it being 10 to 15 years old. There's also a lot of misinformation as cancers are so very different. So please learn with me as I get the information. I'll explain it in very simplistic terms and apologies to my medical friends, as it's very simplistic. Please message me directly for any questions, too. Questions can help me learn.*
>
> *So, the biggest difference between breast cancer and other types of cancer is that breast cancer can be fed by hormones. Mine is progesterone and oestrogen-receptive and HER2-negative, which is the most common and I guess the best to treat. So, the theory is, to be able to stop the hormones, you cut off the supply of food to it and then I also take a tablet that mops up any extra hormones that may be generated by other organs. Then we try*

*to get the immune system, through immunotherapy, to fight the replication of more cancer cells. The drug is state-of-the art and fresh from trials, only ever been used in the last few years, with amazing results and with few experiencing advancements of the cancer. I'm fortunate to be a prime candidate and to access this through the PBS. I'm throwing everything at this and determined to live long, well and help the doctors lift their step significantly. There is no alternative in my mind.*

*I welcome those similar stories of defying the odds just to keep my mind strong. Everything I will do will have a sound basis in science as well, as I believe it takes more than one treatment to do this well. I still have zero symptoms of the cancer even being inside me, despite multiple needles being shoved in my boobs and liver and I've had zero side effects to the drugs and treatment. I'm on a plant-based diet to reduce pressure on my liver while still getting micronutrients. I'm doing acupuncture, infrared, cold therapy, hyperbaric oxygen, and infusions of vitamins. I'm the fittest I've ever been and plan to stay that way. So, spin, personal training and ballet continue.*

*Breath work and some TLC and emotional healing go without saying, too. I cannot express how I feel so supported and loved by everyone right now. You've all kept my family hugged and strong. The messages, calls, flowers, cards, gifts, meals, hugs and visits all mean so much. Even when I've been slow to reply or sometimes don't know what to say, thank you for being there. It's honestly made all the difference over these last few months.*

The reception of my news and the narrative by my friends and family has been nothing short of incredible. Their response has been filled with an outpouring of support, love, and strength. From the moment I shared my diagnosis, they have embraced me with open arms and surrounded my family with unwavering care. The messages, calls, flowers, cards, gifts, and meals have meant the world to me, serving as constant reminders that I am not alone in this journey. Even during times when I may have been slow to reply or struggled to find the right words, their presence has made all the difference. The overwhelming support and love I have received have kept my spirits high and my family uplifted.

Once you are in a strong position, once you have constructed your own narrative and the approach you will take, you can use your communication skills as you become your own PR manager.

You may feel that communication is not always the most important factor in achieving success. You may believe that while effective communication can be helpful, other factors—such as experience and medical knowledge—are more critical in determining success. Or you may feel that communication skills are innate and cannot be learned or improved.

But communication is a learned skill that we can constantly enhance and refine. We teach this to children, but as adults, we tend to become complacent about the power of the words we use to communicate. My earlier example of the shaping power of name-calling in the schoolyard and its equivalents in our adult lives show we have all experienced, at a fundamental level, the power of words and what they communicate.

You might start by constructing your own message about your cancer. You might choose to disseminate it, as I disseminated mine, by means of social media, or you could use a text message or even a letter to a friend. This can be an empowering step in building your new narrative.

Any significant change or transformation will involve the natural response to loss that is grief. You might grieve, for example, the loss of the way things used to be, the loss of a particular individual or relationship, the loss of a job, even the loss of a familiar routine. Equally, even as you let plans go and embrace the unknown, you might grieve the plans you had laid out for your future, your vision of how your life would play out.

For all that your experience of what is lost may result in feelings of disappointment and frustration and fear of what lies ahead it is also, as any counsellor could tell you, an opportunity for growth, learning, and new beginnings.

I grieved for a long time. I think back now to the night I discovered the indentation on my boob. You'll remember I had just sent my kids a text and a goodnight kiss together with a selfie of me in my bubble bath before I headed out for some fun after a busy, beautiful few days in Melbourne. Every time I look at that photo, I think to myself, "Goodness, in just a few hours, I would see that change in my boob and from there, everything would seem like a bad dream." These were the last hours of life as I knew it and they were so good.

Everything changed. My big plans for how my life would unfold after what had been tough few years were scuttled. I said to a friend, "It feels like suddenly others perceived me differently and imposed a new identity on me and yet inside, all I feel is the same old me. I am the same person who sat in that bubble bath, but I'm just facing a new life challenge, and this is a life challenge." I will be me, "the same old me," for a very long time.

The narrative around cancer or, as I prefer to call it, the inflammatory illness, is debilitating not just at a physical level but to your sense of self and identity. It was a kind of identity dysmorphia and in its way it was far more debilitating than any illness or treatment. In the context of cancer, identity dysmorphia refers to the distorted perception or disruption of one's sense of self, body image, and identity following a cancer diagnosis and treatment. Identity dysmorphia in relation to cancer involves feelings of disconnect, dissatisfaction, or distress related to these changes, leading to a distorted view of one's body and identity. I had no physical symptoms or side effects of the disease, yet the side effects as far as my life were incredibly weighty. When you confront a serious illness, it can be a wake-up call that helps us gain a new perspective on our lives and priorities. You may become more aware of what truly matters to you, and you might find new strength and resilience as you face the challenges ahead. You may find you can let go of fear and embrace life more fully than you have in the past. You may become more willing to take risks, to try new things and to appreciate the beauty and wonder of the world around you. I suddenly saw life in colour.

Facing a health crisis may also teach the importance of gratitude and appreciation. You may feel grateful for the support and care of your loved ones and learn anew to appreciate simple pleasures and joys. An illness can be a powerful reminder to live with courage and gratitude, to focus on what's truly important, to embrace life with strength and resilience, and to cherish every moment.

You might be thinking you just want things back the way they were. I spent nights agonising over this—I get it. I wish that were a possibility, but it's not. Fighting or resisting the grief process that is an essential part of letting go of the past will only prolong and intensify your emotional pain and make it even more difficult for you to move forward. When we resist the grief process, we risk becoming stuck in feelings of denial or anger and we may struggle to find acceptance and peace.

Over time, I was able to accept my diagnosis. I don't believe I will ever become accepting of my prognosis, but I have come to terms with it. Grief is a process that involves a range of emotions. Taking care of yourself physically and emotionally can help you cope—small things like getting enough sleep, eating well, exercising regularly, and engaging in activities in which you find joy or relaxation. Talking to others who have experienced similar losses or seeking support from a therapist or support group can be helpful in processing grief and you will feel less alone. Practising mindfulness, of being present in the moment, can help you cultivate a sense of acceptance and peace in the midst of pain.

Mindfulness is defined by the Oxford Dictionary: "a mental state achieved by focusing one's awareness on the present moment, while calmly acknowledging and accepting one's feelings, thoughts, and bodily sensations, used as a therapeutic technique."

I know you might feel as though you're failing when it all gets on top of you—I did. But grief is a process that takes time, and that time will vary from individual to individual. Be patient with yourself and allow yourself the time and space to grieve in your own way.

In this chapter, you've learned how labels can turn into identities and have a profound impact on your mental health, leading to a crisis of confidence. However, by recognising that what you are experiencing is a process of transformation that can be a positive and empowering experience, you will create a mindset that will allow you to rebuild. Please stop thinking the phase you are going through will last forever. It's just part of a process you might liken to the metamorphosis of a caterpillar into a butterfly. You'll reach a place of acceptance by learning to understand the role of communication and developing your own communication skills.

In the next chapter, I will show you the steps and tools that helped me to reframe my crisis.

Chapter Six

# My Reframe

***"Step out of the history that is holding you back. Step into the new story you are willing to create."***

**— Oprah Winfrey.**

The reframe method is a systematic, step-by-step approach to managing your health crisis. It's all about taking steps, strategising and taking action in order to deal with an unforeseen situation in an orderly and structured manner. It's about developing positive and adaptive coping strategies. It is a plan of action borrowed from crisis management theory and practice. The crisis is first broken down into manageable steps, each of which can be addressed appropriately and in turn. The method also encourages you to challenge negative thoughts and beliefs that may exacerbate the crisis at the same time as you develop more positive ways of coping, starting with using better communication skills, with yourself as well as with others.

The reframe method will enable you to feel more in control and empowered to handle the crisis and you may well find you are stronger and more resilient than you thought you were.

How often do you hear people talking about empowering women and creating resilient women? But how often do those same people actually tell you how to do it? The reframe method explains how you can empower yourself to better navigate a crisis and become stronger. It's about using language to calm your nervous system so you can think clearly and make better, stronger decisions to benefit your wellbeing.

Reframing a personal crisis involves finding the words that will enable you to take a new perspective on the way you think about it. Here are some simple initial steps. Acknowledge your emotions. Accept and recognise their presence without judgement or criticism. Allow yourself to experience your emotions, feel them. Experiencing emotion is a normal and important part of the human experience and acknowledging that can help you better understand yourself and others.

Be mindful of your thoughts and feelings. Pay attention to the physical sensations you are experiencing in your body and notice any changes in mood and energy levels. Recognise and acknowledge the thoughts and beliefs that may underlie your emotions. For example, if you're feeling anxious, you may notice that you're having negative thoughts about what's ahead for you. Understanding the cause of your anxiety is a step towards addressing it.

Begin by asking yourself whether your negative thoughts are justified. Is there any evidence to support them? Might looking at your situation from another perspective be more positive and empowering? Might your crisis offer hope, or an opportunity such as personal growth? Might it offer a chance for you to learn new things?

Act on this new perspective. Make a plan to move forward and then take steps to implement it. Taking control is empowering.

Reframing a personal crisis is not always easy but it can be a powerful tool for building growth and resilience, for transformation. With practice, you will learn to see challenges, no matter how overwhelming, as opportunities.

As I faced my breast cancer crisis, I intuitively turned to what I have learned about crisis management in my professional career. Because it helped me, I would like to share it with you. Having a roadmap allowed me to view the long journey ahead one move at a time. It's natural to be overwhelmed in the first stages of a crisis, but a clear and structured strategy, and a good map, will allow you to plan the way forward.

Because you may be unfamiliar with the concept of reframing and how it's used to manage emotions and make better decisions, I will lay out the process, step by step. Think of it as a practical tool, a set of mapping techniques you can use in your everyday life.

As I have confessed, when I was first diagnosed, I was filled with fear and uncertainty. My world was turned upside down and I didn't know how to cope. I felt as though my life was over before it had begun. But I came to see things differently. I realised I had an opportunity to approach my diagnosis in a way that was positive.

What steps did I take to reframe my diagnosis?

- Instead of seeing it as a tragedy, I viewed it as a chance to make positive changes in my life. I focused on the things I could control, like diet, exercise, and self-care routines. I learned to appreciate the small things I had come to take for granted.
- I sought support from loved ones and from a strong team of healthcare professionals. This allowed me to see that I wasn't alone, that there were people who would help me navigate this difficult time.
- I discovered the transformative power of good communication. Through open and proactive dialogue with the forward-thinking medical team I chose to guide me, I found solace amidst uncertainty and anxiety. While the outcome of cancer treatment cannot always be predicted, advancements in targeted therapies, immunotherapies, and precision medicine have revolutionised cancer care, enabling personalised treatment plans based on individual needs. With improved imaging, diagnostics, and early detection, patients now experience better outcomes and enhanced quality of life. These advancements in-still hope for the future, offering a brighter outlook for cancer

> patients and their families. By collaborating with my healthcare professionals, we fostered an environment of positivity and forward thinking, empowering me with confidence on my journey.

The process of reframing allowed me to see my diagnosis as less dark as it offered me an opportunity for growth and transformation. I learned to focus on the present moment and to appreciate the beauty of life, even in the face of adversity. I have learned the importance of resilience, self-love, and community support. My journey through that first phase was difficult, but I am grateful for the opportunity to have learned and grown from it.

An exercise that I would like you to do is to start by being kind to yourself. This might run counter to the way you normally behave but pay yourself a genuine compliment. Think about your best qualities. What are they? Write them down. Firstly, you need to respect and love yourself. You may find this exercise uncomfortable, but it's essential to your wellbeing. Place your hand on your heart and feel it beat. Feel the energy and think about how amazing your body is. You'll have valued yourself and your life in one simple activity. And it's another step to a life-changing reframing of your mindset so that you can recognise challenges as opportunities for growth and transformation. My journey with breast cancer began with uncertainty and fear that left me feeling powerless and vulnerable. But by reframing my mindset, I empowered myself so that I could hope.

- I acknowledged and accepted my emotions, to let myself experience them without self-judgement or criticism. It was scary to face my fears head-on, but it enabled me to understand what was happening to me.
- I was mindful of my thoughts and feelings I learned not only to pay close attention to the physical sensations in my body but also to recognise a set of unacknowledged underlying negative thoughts and beliefs that were making my situation seem worse. It was time for me to challenge them and find alternative perspectives that were more positive and empowering.
- I then acted. I found hope and opportunity by seeking the support and resources I needed. I joined a support group, talked to a therapist, and practised self-care through meditation, exercise, and other activities. Through these actions I discovered a new sense of strength and resilience.

Reframing your mindset is not straightforward but it is transformative. With practice and the support of loved ones and healthcare professionals, you too can find hope and opportunity amidst the challenges of a cancer diagnosis.

As a cancer patient or loved one, you know all too well that battling cancer is not just a physical fight, but also a mental one. The constant stress and anxiety that comes with the diagnosis and treatment can take a significant toll on your emotional and mental wellbeing. When you are diagnosed, your sympathetic nervous system can activate your body's fight or flight response, leading to physical symptoms that can cause even more distress. You may feel exhausted, nauseous, unable to sleep well, which can exacerbate the emotional turmoil you're already experiencing.

What's more, cancer and its treatments can weaken your immune system, leaving you vulnerable to other illnesses and infections which can of course lead to further physical symptoms and anxiety.

It's essential to acknowledge and address the mental as well as they physical battle you're facing. You can take steps to actively manage stress using techniques like meditation, mindfulness, and yoga, all of which can help activate the parasympathetic nervous system and counteract the stress response of the sympathetic nervous system. You will be acting positively to improve your physical and mental health outcomes and your quality of life by maintaining your resilience.

As someone who has faced a breast cancer diagnosis, I understand firsthand the negative emotions and stigma that come with it. The label "cancer patient" can, in itself, be overwhelming and daunting, but instead of seeing cancer as a sentence or something to be ashamed of, I chose to view it as a chronic illness that would impact my life but not define it. By reframing my mindset, I came to see myself as a warrior, someone who was facing a challenge head-on and taking control of my health and wellbeing. This change in my outlook enabled me to take a more optimistic and active approach to my care, resulting in a higher quality of life beyond my cancer diagnosis.

Soon after my diagnosis and in the month before my first scans, I was packing my bags for a trip to LA. Doubts crept into my mind. The idea of overseas travel felt daunting. The negative media articles I read about breast cancer added to my anxiety and I doubted whether I had the physical and mental stamina I'd need. But I refused to let my doubts and fears hold me back. Little did I know, this trip would become a testament to my strength and resilience and a reminder of the power of the mind.

One of my most memorable experiences is completing the three-hour hike to the Hollywood sign. It was 3 months since I had been diagnosed. On the morning of the hike, I woke up to yet another negative article about breast cancer in the media. It deflated my mood, but I set out and found the strength to keep going. My mind kicked my body into another gear, reminding me the brain is the strongest organ in the body and that it programs everything, every cell, every thought. I wanted to remember this climb and the feeling of being on top of the world, both physically and mentally. It was a reminder that even when faced with doubt and negativity, I have the power within me to push through and accomplish anything.

Escapism can be a positive way to reconnect with yourself after a diagnosis of breast cancer. When I went to LA, I felt I could finally let go of my worries and just be myself again. The warm sunshine in Palm Springs, the vibrant energy of Melrose Avenue, and the breathtaking beauty of Beverly Hills helped me to feel alive and free once more. For a moment, I could forget my diagnosis and just enjoy the present. I felt I was reconnecting with the person I used to be before cancer, and it was wonderful. Escapism needn't be just about ignoring or denying reality. It can be about giving yourself a break and reminding yourself of the beauty and joy that still exists in the world.

Looking after yourself, including taking the time to escape for a while, is crucial not only for your own wellbeing but also for those around you— especially children, if you have them. Children are always watching and learning from their parents, so it's important to set a positive example. By showing your children that it's okay to prioritise your own self-care and mental health, you are teaching them the value of self-love and the importance of taking time to recharge and rejuvenate.

I wanted my trip to LA to send a message to my children that it's important to embrace life and all it has to offer, even in the face of adversity. I wanted to show them we can choose to live our lives with joy and passion, even when things get tough. By taking the time to focus on myself and my wellbeing, I would come home refreshed, energised, and ready to be the best version of myself for my children and those around me.

When I look back on my journey with breast cancer, I am grateful for the love I developed for myself along the way. Facing difficulties taught me to value and appreciate myself in ways I had not before. This newfound love for myself led to a newfound confidence and a newfound sense of sexiness. It's amazing how loving and accepting yourself can change your entire demeanour and outlook on life. During my trip to LA, I was my best self, radiating confidence and joy. Escaping from the stresses of daily life allowed me to reconnect with myself, and it was a truly transformative experience. I will always remember how I felt during that trip, and I will always strive to love and appreciate myself.

To sum up, acknowledging the difficult emotions and mental strain that come with cancer, and taking action to manage them, can improve your overall health and wellbeing. A part of this is knowing you are not alone in this battle, and that there are resources available to help you navigate the mental and emotional challenges of cancer.

You might be wondering whether you need to take this particular step. It's important to understand it is part of your journey, and will, at some level, occur anyway. But acting consciously will help you find more meaning in your crisis. Think back to a challenging time and what you learned from it. Are there aspects that you are proud of? Consciously learning from earlier experiences is part of that reframing.

You may not be ready, and this is okay. Take this at your pace. It's your crisis, and it's your life. You matter. You can use this process to examine what is occurring around you and find meaning, even in the midst of feeling depressed or hopeless.

You may be at a crossroads but remember that truly living will come with the exhilaration associated with a feeling of risk. It may be challenging, but to be brave is empowering. Life is short, and it's important to make the most of the time you have, especially after facing a life-threatening crisis like cancer. It's easy to get caught up in the past and what could have been, but the only moment we have is now. Choosing to embrace a new life can be a way to let go of the past, shed old beliefs and behaviours that no longer serve us, and move forward with renewed purpose and meaning. It takes courage to step into the unknown, but the rewards are immeasurable. By choosing to create a new life, you will open yourself up to new possibilities for growth, connection, and joy. It's a reminder that we all have the power to shape our own lives, and that ultimately our journeys are in our own hands. So, take a deep breath, have faith in yourself, and step into the unknown with an open heart and mind. You never know what wonderful surprises life has in store for you.

I've shown you how I reframed my crisis. I hope you can take some positives from my experience to apply to your journey. It's now time to rebuild the personal brand that is you. The next chapter outlines the process through which you will look at all aspects of your life from the way you live, work and love to your mindset for your new life. It's new beginnings time.

# Chapter Seven

# You Can Do It Too: My Journey and Tips

***"The future belongs to those who believe in the beauty of their dreams."***

**- Eleanor Roosevelt.**

Right now, you might be feeling your world is falling apart. You can't believe the reality of your diagnosis or the impact it's going to have. You feel panicked, scared and, to a degree, you grieve the life you once had. I felt all of that and I won't lie—it wasn't easy. It took me fully 90 days to reach a place of acceptance that allowed me to see clearly and imagine into existence a framework for how my life was going to be.

I looked at it as I would any brand-rebuilding business. I asked myself, "What do I value, moving forward?" I needed to make a shift. I needed to value myself. I had always put others first, prioritised others' feelings, needs, and wants over my own. I was a people pleaser, always afraid to say no. This changed in an instant. Suddenly, my life was the most important thing, and I would do anything to hang onto it.

Cancer fast-tracked a mindset shift I had long needed. I wished I'd been able to make the shift without the cancer but given I couldn't change that; how could I make the most of my life? I came to realise how often I'd allowed my life to be shaped by what was happening in others' lives. I decided to simplify my life, and this became a key theme and value for me moving forward.

Just as a business facing a crisis can benefit from breaking down their operations and planning, I carefully dissected and considered each aspect of my life. I broke my daily life down into its various components and thought carefully about each one—my work, my parenting, managing my wellness and health, deciding where and how I wanted to live.

I've done a lot of reading around the impact of stress and on people suffering from cancer. Of course, I'm not a medical expert, but I am aware of research that suggests they have the potential not only to exacerbate but even to cause cancer. It is clear that stress is damaging to physical as well mental health, whether directly or indirectly, so anything you can do to eliminate it from your life, or at least reduce it, will be beneficial.

Simplifying my life and engaging in mindfulness activities became pivotal in reducing my stress. As I started to prioritise what truly mattered and let go of unnecessary clutter, I found a sense of calm and clarity. It was like a breath of fresh air in the chaos of daily life.

One of the mindfulness practices that had a profound impact was breath work. Taking moments to focus on my breath and breathe intentionally allowed me to activate my body's relaxation response. With each inhale and exhale, I could feel the tension melting away, leaving me feeling more at ease and centred. It became a simple yet powerful tool for managing stress in the midst of a hectic day.

Another practice that brought me solace was journaling. I would pour my thoughts, emotions, and experiences onto the pages of my journal. It was a safe space for me to express myself, reflect on my feelings, and gain insights into my own journey. The act of writing itself felt liberating, helping me release pent-up stress and providing a fresh perspective on challenges.

Nature became my sanctuary. I made it a point to spend time outdoors, immersing myself in the beauty of the natural world. Whether it was taking a walk in the park, sitting by a serene lake, or simply appreciating the vibrant colours of a sunset, connecting with nature was a balm for my soul. The tranquillity of those moments and the awe-inspiring sights helped me shift my focus away from stressors, grounding me in the present and restoring a sense of peace within.

I embraced the power of regular exercise. Engaging in physical activities that I enjoyed, like yoga or dancing, became a way for me to release tension and boost my mood. The rush of endorphins and the sense of accomplishment that came with each workout session revitalised both my body and mind. It became a cherished ritual of self-care, allowing me to channel my energy into something positive and invigorating.

This book is an example of the truthfulness and honesty I wanted to share. I wanted to be open. I wanted to express my emotions and feelings. If I was sad, I wanted to cry. If I was happy, I wanted to laugh. I wanted to experience life in colour and in all its highs and lows. I sat one night staring at the television, considering all these things, and I became stuck on, "How do I start?" The next day. I took a piece of paper and wrote down what my next day would look like. This was the beginning of my road map. I broke it down into my work, my family, my wellness. I wrote down all the things I needed to do the next day to fulfil my responsibilities to all the aspects of life that had existed for me in the past and that I would carry with me into the future.

It was raw. It was based on what my life used to look like. When I saw my life in a page it was chaotic and messy. I got a pen, and I eliminated things. "What do I actually need to do? What do I need to do for myself? What do I want to do with the time remaining in my schedule?" My daily schedule turned into a weekly, then a fortnightly, and then a monthly schedule. Then I began to schedule what my next year would look like. What were my goals? What were some things I wanted to achieve?

Through this process, I came to recognise what I valued. My goals were not material; they were based around experiences, feelings, emotions, and moments of joy—things I could look forward to, things I could look back on, things I could share with people and things that would give me a feeling of accomplishment and fulfilment.

You may not yet feel you've reached a point of acceptance or a point from which you can plan, but please trust this process. Taking the first steps towards recognising what you value and how your life might look may help you reach the point of acceptance—a that's a win. You may gain a sense of fulfilment that you're achieving something and that's another win. Celebrate those wins.

I was living well with cancer and it seemed to be receptive to treatment. My work and my career were important to me, and I decided I wanted to keep them. However, I needed to rationalise my work and life balance. I needed to work out what areas of my work I enjoyed most, the people I wanted to work with, and how I could pivot aspects of my business and career to work in with my new life schedule.

I had conversations with the people I worked with, sharing my vision of how I wanted things to be. I re-crafted some of the marketing around my business and, step by step, I attracted the clients, the business and the projects that were right for me. It was amazing to see my vision reflected in my actions and to be rewarded with positive responses.

I worked smarter, not harder. I shortened my workdays, and I powered through those hours whereas before I had been working longer but not all the time spent was focussed. I built into my schedule time with my children, time for exercise, time for cooking, time for reading, time to just "stand and stare"—and those became my rewards. I would power through a few hours, then have some time to reflect, smell the roses and just enjoy a few moments to myself. This became a healthy pattern, and with time I felt that I could take on more and more on without jeopardising my health.

Through my cancer journey, I saw the impact and my value from special people around me–my children, my family, and my close friends. Being able to see that, and to feel that value, triggered a response. I wanted to enjoy and spend more time—quality time—with them. I planned my afternoons so that when my children came home, we could just be together—no work, no phone, no devices, just one-on-one. I enjoyed surprising them with baked treats when they came in from school and I loved seeing the looks on their faces when they saw how much I'd been looking forward to seeing them. Having those conversations after school and leaning into what was happening in their world brought joy to everyone.

I planned holidays for our family. I didn't care where we stayed. The packing and organising that used to annoy me ceased to be a bother. I enjoyed the beautiful anticipation of being at a beach, going on an adventure, or even going away for a night to see a show. We craved these escapes and they allowed me to feel I was giving back to my kids. They were having to manage their own emotions and responses to my illness, and I wanted us all to have some shared time, shared therapy.

The more vulnerable I became, the more I noticed those around me opening up and revealing their own vulnerabilities. It was a beautiful thing to see. One night on a family holiday, I was sitting with my parents, my sister, her partner, my nieces and nephews, my extended family, nieces, and nephews, and my own children. One of my nephews opened up about challenges he was facing, and he openly expressed emotion. Like me, he felt safe, surrounded by love. A problem shared is a problem halved, as they say. I felt so proud of him, but also proud of our family and proud of myself. I saw how I could be a powerful positive influence on others. That moment remains etched in my memory. It reminded me of the unique bond we share as a family, and the incredible strength that comes from opening our hearts to one another. Each and every one of those kids is special, and I'm grateful that we've cultivated a connection built on honesty and acceptance. It's a precious gift that continues to shape our lives in the most beautiful ways.

I have parented differently since my diagnosis. I remember someone telling me it's almost as though you fast-track your kids' lives because they may need to be grown up and independent and not need you too much. To a degree, that's true, but the way I look at it is I simply want them to get the most value out of me as their mother. I take moments to show them things, to talk about things, and to prepare them for life in different ways. Every experience and every moment we have together is an opportunity. I make the most of it. Being their mother is a magnificent gift.

I had always taken my children away for one-on-one time, nights away and special adventures. But since my diagnosis there's been a change. I talk to them about life—their hopes and their dreams as well as what scares them. I ask whether there is anything they want to talk about? I ask what is happening in their world? I feel I have come to know them as I hadn't known them before. There are moments when I feel I am more than their mother. I feel at one with them.

As I embarked on this new chapter of life, it was as if a veil had been lifted from my eyes. I began to see my children not just as extensions of myself, but as unique individuals with their own vibrant characters. I marvelled at their quirks, their passions, and the little details that made them who they were. Every conversation, every laugh, and even every tear became treasures to cherish. My diagnosis taught me the invaluable lesson of being fully present and appreciating the beauty of my children's souls. In their innocent presence, I found solace, joy, and a profound love that fuelled my determination to create meaningful memories and nurture their growth every step of the way.

My daughter is a strong, determined, driven young woman with a wicked sense of humour. She's an old soul and has been here before. She gets things, people, situations. She has the gentlest heart. She loves children, especially little ones she can scoop up, cuddle, and play with. She's attentive. She'll make the most beautiful mother one day. She has extraordinary academic and business gifts. She's brilliant, always achieving top grades and excelling in everything she does. But what sets her apart is her warm, caring nature and her ability to connect with others. She has a natural talent for building relationships, making people feel at ease, and truly understanding their needs. Her creativity is awe-inspiring, and she always finds new ways to innovate and push boundaries. Watching her grow into a well-rounded and accomplished young woman is a source of immense pride and joy for me. I can't wait to see all the amazing things she will accomplish in the future with her unique blend of skills and talents. When we shop together, I am no longer just shopping. I watch the things she is drawn to—the colours, the styles. I watch her try things on and realise that she is growing into a remarkable young woman who is making her way in the world. We shop, we go to a show, we hang out, we go for walks, we belly laugh, and we have some special moments. She once told me through tears that I am important to her and what I mean to her. I showed her how important she is to me and how much I love her.

When my old friends spend time with my daughter, I watch my past and present connect. As my friends and I recall on old times, I see my daughter's eyes light up. I love to see her seeing the person her mum used to be, and how that person has evolved to become the woman she knows. It lets me realise my old life and my current one is not so different after all, and that the values and experiences I gained in my past are still very much a part of who I am now. I am reminded that our past is a part of us, and that the people we have shared that past with continue to shape and influence us in meaningful ways.

My son is younger. He is an exceptional young man with a heart of gold. His imagination and insatiable curiosity drive him to explore and learn about the world around him. His intelligence is undeniable, and he has a way with words beyond his years. He is a natural-born writer and storyteller, with a gift for weaving words together in a way that captivates and inspires. He also has a talent for sports and enjoys being active, but his true passion lies in his creativity and his ability to think deeply about complex topics. His emotional intelligence and sensitivity make him a compassionate friend and a natural leader who brings people together. He is a well-rounded and unique individual with a bright future ahead of him. The adventures we went on together often involved aeroplanes. We always speak to the ground staff and through friends he has had some incredible opportunities, siting in cockpits, meeting pilots and helping flight attendants. He beams from ear to ear and his eyes almost explode out of their sockets. I see on his face the desire to be a pilot or a flight attendant. The energy is palpable.

Together we have wandered the streets, had adventures, visited zoos, and just hung out. He has taken me out for dinner, and we have had dinner party conversations about things like refugee policy, the environment, how he sees the world, things that he thinks could be fixed and, of course, his hobbies, passions, and interests. I just let him chat. He loves to chat, and he's someone that people will always love to chat with. He has a powerful intellect alongside a way of looking at the world that is innocent, forgiving, and full of gratitude. Like his sister, he has a sense of humour. He once paid me the enormous compliment that some of those days we spent together were the best of his life.

My son travelled with me to Sydney while I was there for work. The trip was a great experience for both of us. He saw where I work and the people I interact with daily. He glimpsed the life I live when I'm not at home, the environment I navigate every day, the hustle and bustle of the city. For me, it was an opportunity to share a part of myself he may not have understood before. Seeing him in that environment made me feel incredibly proud, knowing that he was developing an understanding of the world outside our small community. It was a chance for him to see that the world is full of different people, cultures, and experiences, and that his mom is a part of that. It was a bonding experience for us, and I am grateful to have been able to share this part of my life with him.

I tell them both every morning as I give them cuddles how important they are to me, what beautiful humans they are and how much I love them. I have done this every day since they were born and it's how I will start every day for the rest of my life. Whether we are together or apart, I'll find a way.

If you are a mother or an aunt or if you have friends with children, you are close to, what I have said might be a little overwhelming. Don't dwell on it; just take some small steps to move forward in this space. Trust the process and it will become easier day by day. Remember, it took me 90 days to feel at ease and it may take time for you too.

The next step was to look at what I was putting in my body. I'm a staunch believer in controlling what you can and trying not to worry about what you can't. I am fortunate in that early on I had neither symptoms nor side effects. But I knew I needed to keep my body strong in case I became sick. I began with the air I breathed. I'd read much about the effects of oxygen. It's healing and supports our immune system, and it just makes us feel good. I started small with a breath-work teacher and did some intensive sessions. I learned simple techniques to improve the effect of the breaths I took to calm my mind. These helped me ease into meditation until I built it into my daily practice. I'll admit, I haven't perfected it! There are days where I can't set aside the time, but I remind myself that doesn't mean I've failed. I don't give up. I might take a moment in the car before picking up a child. I take five deep breaths, place my hand on my heart to feel my heartbeat and, for those few moments, I'm at one with myself. It's a small step but it can have a massive impact. Don't give up; just keep trying. There's always tomorrow.

Of course, there is more that you can do with oxygen. I tried hyperbaric oxygen chambers and while they worked well for me, oxygen is everywhere and learning how to breathe correctly can help your body absorb it as effectively as possible.

Inflammation is a common issue with cancer. Again, nutrition is a factor. After my diagnosis I decided to go on a largely plant-based diet, customised to include eggs and fish, to reduce inflammation.

The plant-based diet raised my energy levels, cleared my system, and gave me a little more zest in my step. Because I had been raised in the country, it was difficult for me to part with my cherished dairy and meat, yet I took it as a challenge, and I relished trying new recipes for my family. I worked through the things we liked and eliminated things we didn't, but I made sure my body was getting lots of nutrients and micronutrients to support whatever it was going through.

I purified my water and made sure that everything that was going into my body was the best I could source.

We can't always afford the perfect diet, but even taking small steps will have a big impact. I found I needed a lot of taste and flavour in my food, but because I was spending a fortune on herbs and spices, I grew what I could. My time in the garden was not only enjoyable and therapeutic, but I saved money while keeping my taste buds happy.

I occasionally let myself have days off from the diet. For example, if we were on holiday and ate at a wonderful restaurant or if we were in a location where there was a special food, then I'd have a taste. Remember life is still to be lived. Don't punish yourself. Make sure that you continue to enjoy the things you love. I have already referred to the research that points to a deep connection between trauma and cancer. Trauma can affect the body's stress response system, including the sympathetic nervous system and the hypothalamic-pituitary-adrenal (HPA) axis. When you experience trauma, these systems can become dysregulated, leading to chronic inflammation and suppression of the immune system. This inflammation and immune suppression can create an environment that is conducive to the growth and spread of cancer cells. Furthermore, unaddressed trauma can cause ongoing stress and anxiety, which can have a negative impact on your overall well-being. This means it's as crucial to take care of your mental and emotional health after a cancer diagnosis as it is to take care of your physical health, especially if you've experienced trauma. Trauma can result in anxiety, depression, and post-traumatic stress disorder (PTSD), all of which if unaddressed can significantly affect your quality of life and ability to cope with cancer. Taking steps to address trauma through, for example, one-on-one therapy, support groups, or self-care practices, can help you process and heal from earlier experiences as well as what may have been a traumatic diagnosis. Research has found a deep connection between trauma and cancer. It can affect the body's stress response system, including the sympathetic nervous system and the hypothalamic-pituitary-adrenal (HPA) axis. When you experience trauma, these systems can become dysregulated, leading to chronic inflammation and suppression of the immune system. This inflammation and immune suppression can create an environment that is conducive to the growth and spread of cancer cells. I had experienced relationship trauma, fertility struggles, and baby loss before my cancer diagnosis. These experiences had left me feeling helpless and bereft. I was traumatised and this may have contributed to my contracting cancer. Dealing with cancer while also processing past trauma can be challenging and overwhelming. It was important that I recognised the impact on my mental and emotional well-being and that I sought support. Ongoing care of my emotional and mental health is just as important as the care of my physical health in the journey towards healing and recovery.

Even the best relationships can become a source of stress in times of uncertainty Whether you are in a new relationship or in an established one, or whether you are single but looking for a partner, uncertainty about the future can give rise to feelings of self-doubt. You may feel less desirable and even undeserving of love and the fear of rejection that comes with this means you may either risk closing yourself off from your existing partner or resist seeking out a meaningful and fulfilling relationship.

An experience of rejection or abandonment, even when the wound has healed, can leave deep scars that make it hard to value yourself enough to trust a new partner. The first step in building self-esteem and self-love is to recognise that your worth is not determined by external circumstances or by other people's opinions. When you notice yourself indulging in negative self-talk, replace it with positive affirmations that reinforce your worth. Building self-esteem also involves practising self-care and seeking support from loved ones or a therapist to help you navigate the challenges of uncertainty and build resilience in the face of adversity. For help with navigating the challenges of uncertainty, I turned to therapy, support groups, and self-care practices, and slowly I began to heal. It wasn't easy, but I was able to face my trauma head-on and to find the strength and resilience to move forward and regain control of my life.

Remember you are worthy of love and connection, no matter what the future may hold. It takes courage and vulnerability to love yourself in uncertain circumstances, but the rewards are immeasurable. By valuing yourself, you open the door to meaningful and fulfilling relationships that are built on a strong foundation of self-love and self-worth.

Physical exercise has always been an important part of my life, and I cannot stress enough its importance for you. Choose something you love to do, or something you'd love to learn to do, so you remain motivated. Classical ballet is a longstanding joy I wanted to maintain, but a more recent passion is spin class. My spin obsession started during the COVID-19 pandemic when we were all in lockdown. A fantastic spin teacher shot into my life and lit it up like a firecracker. Her zoom sessions got me through some tough times. They gave me something to look forward to each day–a group of people with a shared sense of humour, fun, and vitality. My teacher and many of the people in the class have since become friends and were an important support to me through those first 90 days. Sometimes I knew that when my teacher put on a particular song or talked about the value of gratitude in a motivating way, she was sending a special message to me. Sharing the feeling of exhilaration after a spin session with these amazing people and our amazing teacher is such a gift.

I continued strength training with my personal trainer, with whom I've worked for about five years. He understands that, for me, exercise and training are as much about my mind as my body. He was supportive and encouraging through my diagnosis and he encouraged me to continue to challenge myself in a safe and supportive way. Strength training helped me to feel physically stronger, to test my strength, and to test my endurance. It helped me build the mental capacity to use my mind as well as my body to fight the cancer.

Ever since I was a young adult, I have suffered from endometriosis, along with other women's health issues. During all those past challenges acupuncture has always worked well for me, and I stepped it up a little after my diagnosis. My acupuncturist has become a close and trusted friend and she was with me at every step, explaining the physiological aspects of cancer and the things that we could do to support my body through the treatments.

She also gave me the gift of an incredible meditation about trees and their remarkable resilience. After devastating fires and storms, the forest will regenerate. Not only do new trees appear but survivors adjust, adapt, and grow back to live and thrive. We shared these visions and often I would take photographs of trees that had gone through some form of trauma but bravely showed signs of life. This started a trend of friends sending me similar photos. It became an important vision exercise, something I could think about when I was meditating or doing my breathing exercises. I looked forward to those treatments every few weeks, for both the physical aspect and the emotional support and encouragement she gave me.

In the early stages, I was suffering from joint pain as a side effect of one of my medications. Rather than take yet another pill, I tried infrared saunas or sauna therapy. It had a big impact. It was a way that I could combine my treatment with my meditation, taking some time out, sometimes sharing with a friend or someone else. The physical benefits were remarkable.

The owner of the wellness centre told me about the services and treatments her service offered, and she too became a friend. I could ask questions and gain another view on how I could best support my body. She would send me articles and give me ideas—ways of enhancing treatment that I was having in the saunas and ways that I could rehydrate. It was one more way of feeling loved and supported throughout the journey.

The treatments I received offered me another opportunity to think and speak more positively about my journey. I paid attention to the narrative I was sharing, and I made sure that it was strong, tight, positive, open, vulnerable, sad when it needed to be sad, expressive of my true self.

One of the final steps I took was a practice I put in place in which I paid myself three compliments from the day. I reflected on three positive things about myself, my impact on what happened during the day, so that I could fall asleep feeling not just gratitude for the experiences but grateful for myself. In isolation, it may seem like a small thing, but sleep is one of the most important things when it comes to our good health, both mental and physical. How we fall asleep can affect how we process things in the course of the night and how we will wake up. I can't emphasise this enough. It's part of a natural rhythm but try to enhance it so you can love yourself more.

## Chapter Eight

# My People, My Team

***"Loyalty is what makes us trust. Trust is what makes us stay. Staying is what makes us love, love is what gives us hope, and hope is what makes us truly alive."***

**-— Unknown**

To manage a crisis, such as a breast cancer diagnosis, assembling a reliable team becomes crucial. Every individual will need to determine for themselves who makes up their support system, as it can vary from person to person. In this chapter, I want to share with you the inspiring individuals who formed my team. Beyond the medical professionals, my team also included family members and friends who uplifted me with their unwavering love, understanding, and encouragement. The collective strength and resilience we found through our relationships shaped the outcome of my crisis. Through this chapter, I hope to inspire you to recognise and value the significance of your own team, for it is the power of these connections that can make all the difference in navigating and overcoming any challenge life throws your way.

In the first 24 hours following my diagnosis, I knew I needed my team of family and friends, and I pulled them close. I reached out first to them—and boy, they rallied. My girlfriends called, encouraging me, coaching me, keeping me strong, letting me cry, letting me talk, sometimes giving me tough love. My friends are so important to me. They know me; I know them, and they were just what I needed. There were care packages, flowers, bottles of gin, facials, hugs, gifts of work hours—everything I needed. They rallied and supported my family, too. They hugged my children, cried with my mum, reached out to my sister, and just held us tight.

I can hardly put into words the gratitude I feel for my local and faraway friends who me during my battle. These women, many of whom I had only met later in life, became an integral part of my support system, helping me navigate the toughest time of my life.

Their unwavering dedication was nothing short of incredible. They would drop everything at a moment's notice. They prepared meals with love and care, filling my fridge and freezer with nourishing food that sustained me through my treatment. They gave me treats and funny gifts, and the most gorgeous fluffy blue blanket to snuggle under when I was alone.

But it wasn't just the practical support that made a difference. It was the way they showed up for me emotionally, listening to my fears and anxieties, holding my hand when I needed it most, and reminding me I was loved and cherished.

I cannot express how much their unwavering support and compassion meant to me. We are likeminded women who share our dreams and aspirations, and they were there for me when I needed them most, I will never forget the depth of their kindness, the warmth of their embrace, and the laughter we shared, even during the darkest moments. They are a testament to the power of friendship and community, and I am truly blessed to have them in my life.

But what I love most about both groups of friends is how they make me feel. With my childhood friends, I feel I'm home, surrounded by people who know me inside and out. With my newer friends, I feel anything is possible, and that we can conquer the world together.

Both groups of friends have seen me at my best and my worst, and they still love me for who I am.

I'm so glad I sent those messages telling them I had cancer and needed help. I was at my most vulnerable, but I articulated my need. I know myself. If one of my friends needed me, I would be there in any way I could—and they were there like that for me. While I was fortunate to have friends with medical connections or knowledge who assisted me in assembling my medical team, I understand that not everyone may have access to such resources. However, the valuable lesson I learned from this experience is that building a support network and finding the right team is within reach for everyone, regardless of their personal connections. It may require a proactive approach, seeking recommendations from trusted sources, researching healthcare professionals, and reaching out to support groups or patient advocacy organisations. By actively seeking out individuals who can provide the expertise and guidance you need, you can still gather a team of knowledgeable and compassionate individuals to support you through your journey.

My experience of the immediate support I received from my friends could not contrast more sharply with my encounter with my first medical team. As I have said, it was a dismal fail on every level. On paper and from the PR surrounding breast cancer care, you might have assumed I was with one of the best teams in the country. In reality, although through no fault of their own, they were swamped, understaffed, and under-resourced. The organisation had a bad culture around the treatment of cancer and their program was disjointed. Don't get me started on their poor communication. However, through my networks, I was able to get leads on more positive teams. Not only did they connect me with people who were going through the same experience as I was, they directed me to as people who served on different boards, research committees, and expert organisations. Soon I found myself with a medical team whose culture, approach, and values were focused on my living well.

You may be thinking that it is going to be hard to ask for help and be vulnerable. Start small. You might ask someone to pick up a child. Or begin a conversation with a friend about what you're going through. Step by step, conversation by conversation, you will become stronger, and you'll be rewarded as people respond positively. It's important to accept offers.

People want to feel they can do something, so by accepting help, you're helping them too. It's a shared experience.

I encouraged those around me to be open with other people about what I was experiencing and as a result my networks expanded. Friends are often made at a time for a time, and this was certainly the case for me as I connected with other women coping with serious illnesses

Social media has changed the way we connect, and it has given us the ability to make friends with kindred spirits from all over the world. I have been pleasantly surprised by the comfort and support online friendships have given me, whether it's a kind comment on a post or a private message of encouragement. Even if I never meet them in person, I feel a strong connection and their words of support have lifted me up when I needed it most.

I wanted to meet and connect with women who were living well with breast cancer. I wanted some inspiration. I found many of the online forums and online contacts to be negative and I chose to limit my time with them. Seek out and attract people online who can help to keep you strong, who will inspire you and that you will want to keep close on your journey.

Sometimes you can have conversations with people who are sharing your experience that you can't have with others around you, no matter how close you may be. As much as your friends might try to understand, they simply can't, and that's okay. They will support you in other ways. Build your people and your teams so you know who to go to for the kind of emotional support you need at a particular time. Responding to this cancer stuff is, as we've discussed throughout the book, as much a mental game as it is a physical one.

The therapy a psychologist provides is expensive and although mine was superb, I thought constantly about how much money I was spending. I discovered I could manage with fewer appointments if I could talk to and lean on friends between visits. Again, this worked both ways. The things I was talking about with friends could be inspiring and resilience-building for them as well as for me. Life's difficulties and the struggle to overcome them are common to all human experience, so sharing them can be a beautiful value exchange.

I know cancer will always be a part of my life, but I also know I have a community to turn to for comfort and advice whenever I need it. I feel blessed to be part of a group of people, some of whom have overcome tremendous adversity. Their experiences have helped me find joy and meaning in life despite this illness.

As women, we often cherish emotional connections and intimacy in our relationships. Building friendships based on trust and loyalty can create a safe and nurturing space where we can share our feelings and experiences, finding validation, understanding, and a sense of belonging. Cultivating deep connections with friends allows them to become trusted confidantes who keep our secrets while offering unwavering support and loyalty. In my own experience, my friends have played these crucial roles in my life. They have not only provided joy and moments of laughter but have also helped me grow personally and professionally. They have offered invaluable advice, encouragement, and support in achieving my goals and pursuing my dreams. To foster such relationships, be open to new connections, invest time and effort in nurturing existing friendships, and prioritise quality over quantity. Engage in meaningful conversations, show genuine care and support, and be a reliable and trustworthy friend. By fostering these connections, you can build a circle of friends who uplift you, celebrate your successes, and walk with you through the challenges of life.

All my relationships and friendships are a valuable and important part of my life. Sharing experiences with friends can be powerful because it allows us to connect with others on a deep level and create memories that can sustain us for a lifetime. When we share, we open ourselves up to new perspectives, ideas, and insights that we may not have considered before. We gain the sense of community and support that can help us navigate difficult times. My Los Angeles hike was an intense experience, but it was having a friend at my side that taught me the value and undeniable power of a shared experience, whether it's a hike to the Hollywood sign or enjoying a meal with loved ones. Losing a friendship can be painful and confusing for a breast cancer sufferer. It's natural to question what you did that resulted in a friend's disappearance from your life, but their absence may be a projection of their own insecurities, fears, and limitations rather than a reflection of anything you did, let alone of you or your worth as a person. It's important to recognise that some people are simply not equipped to handle the uncertainty and emotional intensity of a personal crisis. They may be afraid of saying or doing the wrong thing, or they may feel uncomfortable with the vulnerability triggered by another's crisis. It's important to remember it's not about you. Focus on the people who are there for you, who offer support and encouragement, and who lift you up when you need it the most. And remember that your worth as a person is not defined by the number of friends you have but by the strength and resilience you embody as you navigate life's challenges.

Not all of us are so fortunate as to have living parents, but at a time when everything seemed to be falling apart, I could turn to mine. They were the pillars of strength I could lean on when I faced my diagnosis, and their love and support made all the difference. If you can call on your parents, they can be the ones who remind you of your worth, who lift you up when you feel down, and who hold your hand through the toughest moments. It's not just their words that are important, but also their presence. For me, there is something comforting about having them nearby, knowing that they are there for me no matter what. They give me a sense of safety and security in an uncertain time. Their unwavering love and support help me find the strength to keep fighting and moving forward, one step at a time.

My parents have been my rock through this journey, each with their unique personalities and strengths. My mother is a born grandmother, with a nurturing and loving spirit that makes everyone around her feel at home. She's the kind of person who never stops, always with a can-do attitude and a young soul that belies her age. Her unwavering support and endless positivity have been a guiding light, reminding me that I'm not alone in this battle. My dad, or the man who has been my dad, is a bit of a larrikin with an eccentric world view. But he's always been one of my biggest fans, cheering me on from the sidelines and pushing me to be my best self. His unwavering belief in me has given me the courage to take on the challenge of my diagnosis with my head held high. Together, my parents have been my sounding board, my confidants, and my advocates. They've made a difficult time a little bit easier, and for that, I am endlessly grateful.

The bond that was forged between my sister and me during my crisis is truly special. Her selfless compassion as she gave me her time, energy, was a gift beyond measure. I find it hard to put into words just how much her support meant to me during that difficult time. The simple act of her being there, listening and holding space for me, made all the difference in the world. And it wasn't just the practical things, like driving me to appointments or staying with me while I recovered from tests. Our shared experience brought us closer than we had ever been. It allowed us to put aside our differences and focus on what truly mattered—supporting and caring for each other in a time of need. Through that process, we were able to heal old wounds and build a stronger, more resilient relationship. I am filled with gratitude and know I would not have made it through without her.

When I was diagnosed, I realised the importance of a supportive work environment. It became clear my colleagues were more than just colleagues; they were my friends and my support system. We shared values and a sense of purpose, and that made all the difference. They were there for me every step of the way. Their unwavering support and encouragement gave me the strength and motivation to keep going, and I will always be grateful for their presence in my life. A few months after diagnosis, I was due to speak at a conference at 7:45am. While I was waiting at the airport, having a teary time, and questioning whether I could do it, I sent a text to my partner: "I think I'm too broken and I'm not ready." But he wouldn't let me give up. One of my colleagues met me at the airport gate and never left my side. They knew what was going on for me, though they never raised it. They were there while I took deep breaths, and I did it. I spoke at the conference. I love the stage and I love bringing out the best in others at events. It's something I've loved since my ballet days, so I was in my element. My identity and confidence had been rattled, and it's not until you face the perception of others that you understand the weight this has on you.

That morning, I felt lost. I felt that to stand on that stage would be to expose myself and everyone in that audience would see how I felt. I was so lucky that I was supported by two beautiful men and a beautiful woman I work with who held this space for me. I'll forever be indebted to them for this. I regained my confidence, but I couldn't have done this without those amazing people by my side.

Another memory of friendship I have is from the New Year's Eve following my diagnosis. It was hitting me hard. Everyone was excitedly discussing their resolutions for the new year, and I was reluctant to participate. It was a dear friend who yanked me out of this mindset to say, "Well, my dear, we are all in the same boat. None of us knows what is going to happen tomorrow, next week or next month, and we are still making resolutions. We have hope, and so do you."

I knew that was true. All of us live with uncertainty. Certainty is a myth. Life is like a choose-your-own-adventure novel, and you must pick a direction and go for it. Anything can happen to us at any time. I've now embraced my anxiety but I'm not talking simply about the cancer journey, but the life journey.

I am grateful to my cancer for teaching me this life lesson. I've been given the gift of living my life with the deepest emotions, feelings, and appreciation for the now. I am still anxious, but I'm embracing that in the knowledge that anxiety exists in a state of hope veiled in fear. I can manage the fear just as you can because of that hope and the support of others.

You might be feeling those overwhelming emotions right now. Even as I'm writing this, I have tears streaming down my face, but tears of sadness have been turned into tears of gratitude and love. I'm thinking about all the special people in my life and our shared experiences—good times, bad times, happy times, sad times. I'm thinking of the laughs, the silliness and the funny things that have gone wrong. I'm thinking about dark moments where we've been our most vulnerable together and the profound impact this has had on me as a person and will have on me and my life moving forward.

I cry a lot now. I actually cry a little more than I did when I was first diagnosed. The tears back then expressed sadness entangled with anger, but now I cry tears of joy, tears of happiness. You'll get there too. It might seem overwhelming and unfathomable now, but you will get there.

## Chapter Nine

# Reflection

This book has allowed me to share with you my journey as I adapted the PR crisis management strategies, I have used in my 20-year professional career to navigate the crisis that is a breast cancer diagnosis. I hope that, in the process, I have achieved my aim of providing you with a roadmap for your own journey. I know from experience how easy it is to feel you're at the mercy of your diagnosis, but I'm here to remind you that, like me, you are the CEO of your own life. You now have the tools and the strategies to manage and navigate your crisis with strength and resilience.

Reflection is an important part of managing any crisis and reflecting on mine has helped me to grow and become stronger and more resilient.

I have laid out some ways in which a business model of crisis management can usefully map onto your crisis. When a business faces a crisis, it must take the time not just to reflect on the crisis and why it occurred, but to analyse the strengths and weaknesses of the response. What was most effective? In other words, reflection allows a business to face what has happened, to respond to it positively, and to prepare for future crises should they occur. The business builds a capacity for resilience. You can use reflection similarly as you manage your crisis.

As I was going through my crisis, I found that taking the time to reflect on my experiences aided both my healing and my growth as a person. It allowed me to process the range of emotions I was experiencing—from fear and sadness to anger and frustration. It also helped me to gain valuable insights into:

- what had worked well and continued to work well for me in terms of the treatment I received.
- what could have been done differently.
- what control I had in the process.

Through reflection, I was able to identify patterns and behaviours that aggravated the crisis and to use this knowledge to make changes and improve my response in the future. But perhaps most importantly, reflection allowed me to build resilience. It helped me to identify my coping mechanisms and what helped me to get through the crisis. It also allowed me to identify areas in which I struggled and to make plans to build my resilience further in those areas. I felt more confident and better equipped to handle future challenges, and more confident in my ability to bounce back from adversity.

Reflection is recognised to be a powerful tool for healing and growth and is as essential for personal crisis management as it is for business management. By taking time to reflect on our experiences, we can gain valuable insights, process our emotions, and build resilience. It is a practice that has helped me tremendously, and one that I believe can benefit you.

As I have made clear, no aspect of facing the crisis that is a breast cancer diagnosis is easy. This means that reflection on the process may be emotionally taxing as it will require you to confront some of your deepest fears and vulnerabilities. Reflecting on a crisis can bring up a range of complex emotions, from sadness and grief to anger and frustration. These emotions can be overwhelming, and it can be hard to find the time and energy to address them when so much else is going on. But despite these challenges, reflection remains essential since it will allow you to gain valuable insights into what is happening and, in identifying your strengths and weaknesses, build your capacity for resilience. It is through reflection that you will find healing and growth.

For me, reflection has been a difficult but essential part of my journey. It has allowed me to confront my fears and vulnerabilities, and to acknowledge things I could have done differently. And it has allowed me to find meaning and purpose in my experiences, and to use what I've learned to help others going through similar challenges by writing this book.

It's natural to be hard on yourself in reflection, especially when you're going through a crisis or a difficult experience. You may be overwhelmed by painful feelings that you could have done more or been stronger.

I know from personal experience how challenging it can be to practise self-compassion in reflection. During my own crisis, I found myself constantly dwelling on my mistakes and shortcomings and feeling I had let myself and others down as I responded to my diagnosis. But as I learned the value of self-compassion for healing and growth, I began to treat myself with kindness and understanding. I could acknowledge my mistakes without blaming myself or dwelling on them. And I was able to recognise my strengths and accomplishments and celebrate my resilience and perseverance. I was able to move forward with a renewed sense of purpose and direction, and to use what I had learned to help others going through similar challenges.

While you may find it difficult to overcome self-criticism in reflection, by practising self-compassion, focusing on your strengths, and celebrating your accomplishments, you can learn and grow from your experiences in a way that is empowering and healing.

I use a number of practices and tools as I reflect, some of which you might find helpful.

One simple and very powerful exercise I recommend to you is journaling. Writing down my thoughts and emotions allows me to process my experiences in a safe and private space, and to explore my feelings honestly without fear of judgement or criticism. It also allows me to track my progress and celebrate my achievements, no matter how small.

I also practise mindfulness meditation. By focusing on my breath or on a specific object such as a cloud in the sky or a tree in the street, I find I can stay present and grounded during reflection, even when my thoughts and emotions are overwhelming. I use the technique to manage emotions ranging from anxiety to fear to sadness as I find a sense of calm and clarity in the midst of crisis.

Positive self-talk has been a powerful tool in my reflection process. When I find myself dwelling on my mistakes or shortcomings, I try to shift my focus to my strengths and accomplishments. By reminding myself of my resilience, courage, and achievements, I can bring to bear self-compassion and kindness. A task I was shown and would recommend to you is to list negative thoughts or self-talk and, beside it, write a second list that counters the negative thoughts with positive ones.

Negative thoughts or self-talk can often hinder our growth and well-being. Some common negative thoughts may include:

- "I'm not good enough."
- "I'll never be successful."
- "I can't handle this situation."

To counter these negative thoughts, it can be helpful to create a second list of positive affirmations or counterstatements, such as:

- "I am worthy and capable."
- "Mistakes are opportunities for growth and learning."

- "I have the skills and determination to achieve my goals."
- "I am loved and valued by the people who matter."
- "I have overcome challenges before and can handle whatever comes my way."

By consciously challenging and replacing negative thoughts with positive affirmations, we can reframe our mindset and cultivate a more compassionate and empowering inner dialogue. This exercise of listing negative thoughts and countering them with positive ones can help us build resilience, boost self-esteem, and foster a more optimistic outlook on life.

Ultimately, reflection is a deeply personal and individual process, and what works for one person may not work for another. But by being patient, kind, and compassionate towards yourself, and by using simple techniques such as journaling, mindfulness, and positive self-talk, you can start the process of reflection and gain valuable insights into your experiences.

One of the reflections of the bigger picture of breast cancer for me is that the journey can be one of the most emotionally overwhelming any woman will experience. The moment you hear those words "you have breast cancer," your entire world comes crashing down. It is as though your life is no longer yours to manage. You're at the mercy of your diagnosis.

But what's even more frustrating is the lack of support and resources available to women with breast cancer. Despite the billions of dollars raised globally each year by charities and foundations, patients are still not receiving the care and support they need.

I remember vividly the challenges I faced during my breast cancer diagnosis. It was a time of overwhelming emotions, where I felt lost, scared, and completely alone. The weight of confusion added to my distress as I navigated the sea of misinformation surrounding breast cancer. The prevalent PR myths created a cloud of misconceptions and misunderstandings that seemed to surround me at every turn. One of the most damaging myths I encountered was the belief that breast cancer only affected older women, when approximately 20% of women diagnosed are under the age of 50. I found myself in my forties, facing this battle. It was during this time that I felt the depths of isolation and lack of support.

Despite these challenges, I refused to give up hope. I sought out resources and support, and I found comfort in the voices of women who were taking the journey with me or had taken it before me. It was through these connections that I realised not only the power of community but the need for more and better-targeted resources and support for younger women with breast cancer.

It's time to start breaking down the myths and start investing and targeting funds in a better way and into the aspects of research, development, and support for women with breast cancer that provide practical guidance and tools for managing emotional and psychological alongside physical challenges. Better health outcomes will flow from a more compassionate and supportive healthcare system that truly puts the needs of patients first.

I have learned a great deal about myself from reflecting on my experiences with the crisis of breast cancer. I have discovered that I am stronger and more resilient than I ever imagined, capable of facing even the most daunting challenges with courage and determination. But I have also learned that it's okay to ask for help and to prioritise my own well-being.

During my journey, I have found solace in the connections I made with others, and I have realised the value of social support and community. These connections were a lifeline during my darkest moments, giving me the guidance, comfort, and sense of belonging I needed to keep going. Reflection has also been crucial to my personal growth and resilience. Through self-examination and honest appraisal of my experiences, I have been able to see my strengths and weaknesses, and to develop a deeper understanding of myself and my needs.

Most importantly, my experiences have taught me the importance of advocating for myself and others. I have seen firsthand the power of the myths and misconceptions that surround breast cancer, and the ways in which they can prevent people from receiving the care and support they need. By challenging these myths and advocating for greater awareness and resources, I hope to make a difference for others facing similar challenges. I believe I can make a positive impact in the world. You will too.

The step that inevitably must follow reflection on the things you want to change is indeed daunting, but it is also exciting. On the one hand, it can be difficult to confront areas of our lives in which we need to make changes. On the other hand, it can be empowering to take ownership of our experiences and use them as a catalyst for growth and transformation for yourself and for others.

For me, reflection has been a deeply emotional and personal process. It has forced me to confront my fears and insecurities, and to examine my values and priorities with a critical eye. But it has also opened new possibilities and opportunities and has given me a renewed sense of purpose and direction.

I know the path ahead will not be easy. There will be setbacks, obstacles, and challenges along the way. But I also know that by using reflection as my guide, I will be able to stay true to my values and priorities and continue to grow and evolve as a person.

So, if you feel uncertain or overwhelmed after reflecting, know you are not alone. The next step may be challenging, but it can also be the beginning of a powerful journey of self-discovery and growth. Embrace the possibilities ahead and take those first steps towards achieving the outcomes you desire.

If your personal crisis is not breast cancer, you can still use these strategies, skills, and techniques. As women, we often juggle multiple roles and responsibilities. When a crisis hits, it can become all-consuming. But by applying the crisis management strategies I've shared from business; you can break down the situation and understand what's going on. Then you can address the crisis, one step at a time.

You can recognise the impact on your identity and move forward with confidence. I know this firsthand from my own breast cancer diagnosis. It was a scary and uncertain time, but I turned to the tools and strategies I use in my profession to manage the crisis and regain control.

That is why I have written this book. I realised I had the tools that you might not have, so I decided to share them. Now you can use them to handle whatever curveball life throws your way.

When you become your own CEO, you open yourself up to a richer, sexier, and happier life. You break down the situation you face so that you know what's going on. You feel in control, and you feel confident—and that spills over into every aspect of your life. You'll find yourself making better decisions, taking more risks, and seizing opportunities you may have chosen to avoid before. Let's not forget about the sexier part. When you're in control and confident, you radiate a certain energy that is undeniably attractive. You feel more confident in your own skin and that confidence is a magnet for others and for wonderful opportunities in all aspects of life.

Most importantly, implementing crisis management strategies to personal crises will make you happier. You'll find yourself in a better headspace, free from the anxiety and stress that can come with the uncertainty that accompanies loss of control. You'll be able to face any challenge that comes your way with a sense of calm and clarity.

Embrace uncertainty and change. Trust in the process. Use the tools and strategies that have proven effective in the business world and apply them to your own life. As women, we bring a unique and essential perspective to society. We are caregivers, nurturers, and creators. We have the power to shape the world around us in meaningful ways. Our ability to empathise and connect with others allows us to build bridges and break down barriers. Our strength and resilience in the face of personal crises inspires those around us and encourages them too to persevere in the face of adversity. We are role models, leaders and change makers. Our contribution to society cannot be overstated. Whether we are fighting for equal rights and opportunities, creating art that touches the soul, or raising the next generation of leaders, we are making a difference.

We must embrace our power and strength and continue to inspire others to do the same. We are essential to the fabric of society and have the ability to create a better future. Remember, a happy life starts with you. Focus on building your confidence, taking care of yourself, and radiating positive energy. Keep moving forward even when it feels difficult and trust that your efforts will pay off in the end. Take a deep breath and take that first step. You have everything you need to create the future you deserve—one that is richer, sexier, and happier.

Taking ownership of your life and embracing personal crises can be scary and overwhelming. It's natural to doubt your own abilities but again I'm here to remind you that you have the power to manage and navigate this crisis with strength and resilience. It's important to shift your mindset and recognise your role as your own CEO. Believe in yourself and your agency. Don't be afraid to take ownership of the situation. You are a match for any curveball you may be thrown.

Of course, there'll be moments of uncertainty and fear. It's natural to want to hold onto a sense of control. But it's okay to let go of that control and embrace the unknown. Break down your situation into smaller, manageable steps and focus on what you can control. Every step forward is a victory, and you'll find yourself gaining confidence and strength along the way.

Remember, certainty is a myth. By recognising this and embracing the reality that is uncertainty, we become wiser and stronger in the face of life's challenges. Life will always be full of unexpected twists and turns. We cannot always control or predict the future. But we can learn to accept uncertainty and embrace it as a natural part of the human experience. Life is full of surprises, as they say.

Acceptance allows us to become more adaptable and resilient. We learn to trust ourselves and our ability to handle whatever comes our way. We become wiser in our decision making, recognising that since there are no guarantees in life sometimes the best thing, we can do is to make a decision based on the information we have at that moment.

I invite you, then, to embrace uncertainty, recognising that to do so is, far from being a sign of weakness, is a sign of strength and resilience. Trust in your ability, as I have learned to do, to navigate life's challenges and emerge stronger and wiser. This brings me back to the limiting effects of negative self-talk. It's so easy to fall into a trap of thinking you're not good enough or capable enough, but such thoughts do not serve you well. It's time to challenge them and replace them with positive affirmations that reinforce your power to overcome any obstacle, your power to thrive.

You are strong, you are capable, and you are worthy of creating a richer, sexier, and happier life for yourself. Take this first step with confidence and trust in yourself. You are your CEO, and you have the power to navigate personal crises with strength and resilience. The future is full of possibilities. It's up to you to seize them.

## An invitation to my reader

I'm passionate about empowering women facing the crisis that is breast cancer to take charge of their own lives. I invite you to be part of this movement. Let's connect and create a community of women committed to empowering themselves and each other. Let's share stories and experiences, offer support and encouragement, and celebrate each other's victories. Together we can challenge the status quo and create a world in which a breast cancer diagnosis is recognised head on as the crisis it is but also seen as an opportunity for growth and transformation. Let's inspire each to take leadership of our lives and embrace our power and resilience.

I invite you to join me on this journey. Follow me on social media. Reach out to me with your stories and experiences. Be part of the change we're creating. Let's lift each other up and create a future full of possibility and potential. Remember, you are strong, capable, and worthy of creating a life that is rich, sexy, and happy. Let's do it together.

One of the most important parts of a crisis is the moment of reflection. As I reflect on my own experience of breast cancer, I'm filled with hope for the future—a future in which women facing this disease are empowered to embrace their own strength and resilience, a future in which the challenges they face are seen as opportunities for growth and transformation.

My wish for the world is that we continue to challenge the status quo and create a new paradigm for those facing breast cancer—a paradigm which we are not defined by our illness but by the way we rise to the challenge, in which we lift each other up and provide support and encouragement when and where it's needed most. Let us continue to empower women facing breast cancer to take ownership of their own lives and trust in their own strength and resilience. You may not be able to rely on breast cancer charitable support systems or networks in the medical profession, but let's learn how to modify them so they work for us.

Let's embrace this journey with a spirit of hope and optimism—and inspire others to do the same. Through my own negotiation of the personal crisis that is a breast cancer diagnosis, I discovered a great love for myself and all the aspects of my life. For the first time, I truly, deeply fell in love with myself, recognising my own strength, resilience, and beauty. As I navigated the uncertainty and emotional intensity of my diagnosis, I discovered a new appreciation for the people and the experiences that make up my life. I fell in love with the small things—the warmth of the sun on my skin, the sound of my children's laughter, the beauty of the sunset. Through this journey of self-discovery through personal crisis, I discovered the beauty that existed within me, a beauty I had not seen before. And I saw my own strength and resilience reflected to me in the love and support of those around me.

Their unwavering belief in me and my abilities helped me to see the beauty within myself and to fall in love with it in a way that was transformative and profound. I also fell in love with the big things—the people who supported me and lifted me up, the experiences that brought me joy and fulfilment, the knowledge that I had the power to overcome any obstacle that came my way.

This great love I discovered is not just about me, but about all women facing a personal crisis. It's about recognising our own worth and power, embracing uncertainty and change, and finding beauty and joy amid difficulty. It's about falling in love with ourselves and our lives in a way that is authentic and deeply fulfilling.

As humans, we tend to label people, to put them into neat boxes that we think we can understand and categorise. We do this because it's easier to label someone than to take the time to truly understand and recognise all the complexities that go to make the human experience. But the weight of judgement that comes with these labels can be heavy and damaging. It can lead to misunderstandings, prejudice, and discrimination. It can prevent us from seeing the full beauty and potential of a person, and from recognising the value they bring to the world. The reality is that every human is complex with a unique set of experiences, emotions, and perspectives. We can never fully understand or appreciate this complexity if we are busy labelling and categorising.

My grandfather, my beloved Pop, has been my North Star for how to live and he has been a guiding light and inspiration for the resilience I speak of in this book. He was an extraordinary example of resilience and strength, and his unwavering spirit left an indelible mark on my heart. Pop, who lived through the Great Depression, faced many personal challenges throughout his life but he never let any obstacle defeat him.

He worked hard, loved every day and every person, and found joy in everything.

Pop's unwavering positivity and determination were a constant source of inspiration for me. He taught me the importance of finding joy in even the smallest things and of never giving up, no matter how tough the situation. He was always there to offer a helping hand, a kind word, or a shoulder to lean on. Pop's strength in the face of adversity was a true testament to his character, and I will forever carry his lessons with me.

Although he is no longer with us, Pop's spirit lives on in the memories and lessons he left behind. He showed me that even in the darkest of times, there is always a glimmer of hope, a reason to keep pushing forward. He taught me that resilience is not about merely surviving but thriving in the face of adversity. Pop will always be my North Star, guiding me through difficult times and reminding me of the strength and resilience that lies within us all.

Let us strive to see beauty and potential in every person, recognising we are all unique and valuable in our own way. Let us approach each other with compassion and understanding, seeking to understand the complexities of the human experience rather than simplifying it with labels. By doing so, we will create a world that is more accepting, empathetic, and kind. Together we can create a world in which breast cancer is not something to be feared but something to be faced with courage and determination, something that, with a little luck, we will live with for a long time. Let's make this future a reality, one step at a time.

# Conclusion

**"Every moment is a fresh beginning."**

**— T. S. Eliot**

The decision to end the book here wasn't made lightly. The reality is, each woman's cancer journey will be unique, and the road ahead will be different for everyone. However, the first three months, those initial 90 days, are a common experience for many. It's a period filled with uncertainty, fear, and anxiety, but it can also be a time of discovering newfound strength, resilience, and hope.

As I write these words, I am sitting on Avoca beach on the Central Coast, my mind again triggered and consumed with the fear and uncertainty of the future. Yesterday marked my first set of scans, and in just a few days, I will receive the results that will tell me whether the treatment is working. It is one of many milestones, but I remind myself that is ok, that is life.

On the day of those first scans, I felt a wave of anxiety and fear wash over me as I prepared myself for the worst. This was the moment my family surprised me with the gift of a puppy. Chloe's warm and loving presence is a reminder that amidst the darkness, there will be a glimmer of light and hope. For the next few days, all that matters is that I am surrounded by family, kids, and cousins on this beautiful beach, cherishing every moment of life and all that I am so lucky to have. And as I wake to the sound of kookaburras, snuggled in bed cuddling my youngest, I know that today is a new day, a good day.

As I rolled through the scanner, I listened to my favourite Beyoncé battle song. I visualised myself lying in a hammock, rocked to the sound of gentle waves, and imagined that instead of the machine's lights I was feeling the sun's warm embrace. Scan anxiety can be a heavy burden to carry. It's uncertainty, fear, and dread all rolled into one. But as I have navigated my own journey with cancer, I have come to realise that scan anxiety can be transformed into an opportunity to see my prognosis from another perspective. Instead of focusing on the worst-case scenario, I have learned to embrace the unknown and approach it with curiosity and hope. Each subsequent scan is a chance to learn more about my body, to gain insight into my health, and to make informed decisions about my ongoing treatment. It's a chance to celebrate the moments of joy in life and the things that truly matter. I have, in other words, chosen to reframe my scan anxiety into an opportunity for growth, learning, and hope. And with each subsequent scan, I am reminded of the resilience and strength that lies within us all.

They may not define me, but the words used to deliver my diagnosis in the first 24 hours continue to haunt me. I work constantly on my narrative, reframing my cognitive mindset so that I'm ready face whatever comes my way. This isn't just something people with cancer should do, of course. Life is unpredictable for all of us, and everyone requires the mental and emotional resilience to face crises and emerge stronger.

All we can control is how we choose to live in the present moment. We can choose to savour the simple pleasures of life, to appreciate the beauty around us, and to connect with the people we love. We can choose to focus on the things that truly matter and to let go the things that don't. When we live in the present, we can fully experience the richness of life and embrace all that it has to offer. So, I am going to do my best to treasure the now.

As I look towards the future for cancer, I hold on to the hope that one day it will be just a chronic illness, with precision and holistic treatments available to all. I believe in the power of our society to grow and become more accepting, loving, and inclusive towards those who are facing cancer. I hope for a world where we can unite and work towards a common goal of zero deaths from cancer, where no one has to go through the fear, pain, and uncertainty a cancer diagnosis brings.

To reflect on my journey with cancer and the people who have supported me, I cannot help but feel hopeful. While cancer is a formidable foe, I believe that we have the power to change the way we approach it and the way we support those affected by it. I envision a future in which we prioritise prevention and early detection, in which we dismantle the stigma surrounding cancer, and in which we embrace a more inclusive and compassionate approach to healthcare. During my experience with breast cancer, I have learned that humans are capable of great resilience, strength, and love. And as we continue to support each other, speak out against injustice, and work towards a brighter future, I am confident we will rise above the challenges and emerge stronger.

As I continue my journey of healing, I am learning to explore the deeper parts of myself and address any lingering trauma. It's not always an easy process, but I am finding that the more I lean into it, the more I am able to release the things that have been holding me back. I am beginning to see that healing is not only about my physical body but also about the emotional and spiritual aspects of myself. I am learning to allow myself to feel emotions and experiences I formerly repressed, and I am learning to love and accept myself. As I do this work—and it is work—I am finding a new sense of freedom and empowerment, and a deeper connection to my inner strength and resilience. I am excited about the journey ahead, and all the growth and healing that is yet to come.

I can't help but dream about my future. I want to see my children blossom into adulthood and I want to meet my grandchildren. I want to continue exploring this beautiful world with my friends, going on adventures, and experiencing all that life has to offer. I hope to continue making an impact in my career and helping others in any way that I can.

But above all, I want to be loved and safe. This desire resonates not only for me but for all individuals, with perhaps a particular significance for women. Feeling loved and safe forms the cornerstone upon which she builds her life, relationships, and sense of self. It is a powerful balm that soothes her wounds, the guiding light that illuminates her path, and the refuge she seeks in times of trouble. Authenticity and wholeheartedness are essential; this feeling cannot be fabricated or substituted.

For far too long, I have yearned and searched for this deep sense of love and safety, often feeling it just out of reach. Nevertheless, I hold onto the enduring hope that one day, I will truly experience this profound love, for it will be an extraordinary gift that brings immense fulfillment and peace. In recognising the beautiful dance between the masculine and feminine energies, I believe that the harmony of these forces can create a profound space of love, trust, and security.

And despite the challenges that come with living with an illness, I want to live well for a long time. The reality of my illness only adds to the challenge, yet I am determined to heal and grow and to find beauty in each new day.

A beautiful ballerina friend introduced me to the tale of "The Empty Boat" by Chuang Tzu, in which a man is consumed by rage when he sees a boat drifting aimlessly towards him. He unleashes a torrent of angry words and curses, only to be filled with confusion and embarrassment as the boat comes closer and he realises it is empty. The story is a powerful reminder of how easily we can project our fears and frustrations onto others, even when they are not at fault. It reminds us to take a step back, assess each situation, and not let our emotions take control of us.

By sharing my experiences and reflections on those first 90 days from diagnosis, I hope I have provided a guide and a source of support to others on their cancer journey. And while the road ahead of you may be different from the one, I have travelled, I hope you find something in my experience that might be applied and adapted to whatever challenges you may face.

As I come to the end of this book, I want to express my deepest gratitude to all the people who have supported me on this journey. To my family and loved ones, who have been my rock and my source of strength throughout, I am forever grateful. To my friends and colleagues, who have gone above and beyond to show their love and support, I am blessed to have you in my life. You have shown me my beauty and value, that I matter. To the healthcare professionals who have cared for me with such compassion and expertise, you are true heroes.

And to you, my reader who has joined me on this journey, I want to wish you all the love and support in the world as you navigate your own challenges and triumphs. May you find the strength, resilience, and joy that lives within you, and may you always know that you are loved. Remember, you are capable of great things, and I believe in you.

With all my heart, thank you.

# Acknowledgments

I embarked on the journey of writing this book with a dual purpose in mind. Firstly, my intention was to provide support, guidance, and inspiration to women who are navigating their own breast cancer journeys. I wanted to share my experiences, insights, and lessons learned in the hopes of offering solace and guidance during challenging times. My desire is to empower women to face their own adversities with strength, resilience, and a renewed sense of hope.

Secondly, this book serves as a legacy for my children, a testament to the love and determination that defines our family. By documenting my journey, I aim to leave behind a tangible expression of my experiences, values, and life lessons for them to cherish and learn from. It is my hope that this book will serve as a source of inspiration and guidance for them as they navigate their own paths, providing them with the tools and insights needed to overcome obstacles and thrive.

Additionally, through the creation of this book, I aspire to contribute to the financial well-being of my children's future. The proceeds and impact generated from this book will help support their dreams, aspirations, and provide for their future needs. It is my heartfelt wish that this legacy serves as a lasting tribute to the love and dedication I have for my children, ensuring their well-being and providing opportunities for them to flourish.

In writing this book, I have poured my heart and soul into its pages, hoping to uplift, educate, and inspire. It is my greatest desire that this narrative resonates with readers, offering comfort, motivation, and a sense of connection. Together, let us embrace the power of storytelling to empower others, leaving a legacy of strength, resilience, and hope.

I would like to extend a heartfelt acknowledgment to the many individuals who have played a significant role in the creation of this book. Their unwavering support, love, and presence have been the foundation upon which this project has been built.

First and foremost, I want to express my deepest gratitude to my children, whose unwavering belief in me and unconditional love have been a constant source of inspiration. Your resilience and strength have been a guiding light throughout my journey, and I am grateful for the joy and purpose you bring to my life.

To my parents, thank you for your unwavering support, guidance, and encouragement. Your love and wisdom have been a pillar of strength, and I am forever grateful for the values you have instilled in me.

I am immensely grateful to my family and friends who have held space for me and stood by my side during the most challenging moments. Your unwavering support, understanding, and acts of kindness have given me the strength to persevere. Your presence has been a source of comfort and reassurance, reminding me that I am never alone no matter how lonely the journey may feel.

A special mention goes to my sister and girlfriends, who have been my pillars of strength and sources of solace. Your unwavering support, understanding, and empathy have provided a safe space for me to express my fears, hopes, and dreams. Your friendship and sisterhood have enriched my life in countless ways, and I am grateful for the bond we share. You are my soul mates and true partners in crime!

I want to express my deep appreciation to those who have served as mentors and role models, guiding me through the intricacies of self-discovery and personal growth. Your presence in my life has been a constant source of inspiration, challenging me to dig deeper, expand my boundaries, and unlock my fullest potential. Your teachings have not only shaped my physical well-being but also nurtured my mental, emotional, and spiritual health.

To all those health and wellness inspirations who have shared their expertise, knowledge, and passion with me, thank you for illuminating my path and enriching my journey. Your teachings and guidance have empowered me to make transformative changes and embrace a life of greater health, vitality, and self-awareness.

I would also like to express my gratitude to the healthcare professionals who have been instrumental in my journey. Your expertise, compassion, and dedication have made a profound impact on my well-being, and I am grateful for the care and guidance you have provided.

To my editor and publishing team and amazing assistant, thank you for your dedication, expertise, and commitment to bringing this book to life. Your insights, guidance, and attention to detail have been invaluable in shaping this narrative.

I am deeply appreciative of the organisations, foundations, and support groups that provide resources, advocacy, and support for individuals and families impacted by cancer. Your tireless efforts in raising awareness and offering assistance are truly commendable.

Lastly, to the readers and supporters of this book, thank you for joining me on this journey. Your interest, encouragement, and presence are deeply appreciated. It is my sincere hope that this book resonates with you, offering solace, inspiration, and a sense of connection.

To all those mentioned and the countless others who have contributed in their own unique ways, I am profoundly grateful for your presence in my life. This book would not have been possible without your love, support, and belief in me. Thank you for holding space for me and for being a part of this remarkable journey.

With deepest appreciation,

Danica

www.shehasbreastcancer.com

danica@danicabpr.com

@shehasbreastcancer

Made in the USA
Monee, IL
11 November 2026

68342108R00095